DEATH WISH

TALES FROM Eternity

Liminal Books

Between the Lines Publishing
1769 Lexington Ave N., Ste 286
Roseville, MN 55113
btwnthelines.com

Published: March 2024

Original ISBN (Paperback) 978-1-958901-82-3

Original ISBN (eBook) 978-1-958901-83-0

$\mathscr{D}$EATH $\mathscr{U}$ISH

TALES FROM *Eternity*

Nan Banks

What they are saying…

"None of us can know about the afterlife until we know. This book brings that home and it is a great read. *Death Wish: Tales From Eternity* brings levity to a potentially fraught topic, and I am not aware that any other end-of-life book does that. I expect that Death Wish will appeal to a wide audience, minus hard core atheists and hard-core fundamentalists!"

- Gary Ross-Reynolds, Death Doula, PhD, RN

"This is the book I needed to read … now. I've been thinking a lot about my spiritual practice, being raised Catholic and trying to figure out how it all fits in. *Death Wish: Tales From Eternity* has been an answer to that prayer. I adore the human approach to spirituality and have gained so many insights. Wonderfully written and truly a gift for me, and us all."

-Sharon McIntosh, President, And Then Communications and Coaching

"This book is going to provoke a lot of discussion and controversy! The juxtaposition of humor, the research and the dialogue among the characters brought me to tears on one occasion. Like nothing I've read before! If you liked *The Shack*, you'll love *Death Wish: Tales from Eternity*."

Rev. David Eck, Lutheran Minister

To my parents, Guynell and Albert, who taught me the love of a good story, well-told.

Betty and the "Hooligan"

…and after my body has decayed, yet in my body I
will see God! I will see him for myself. Yes, I will see
him with my own eyes. I am overwhelmed at the
thought!

(Job 19:25–27)

Do not search for God outside of you…His only abode
is in your heart.

Meher Baba

I just died and that's ok. I was so looking forward to
walking past the pearly gates of Heaven, smiling at St. Peter

1

and saying, "Pete, honey, go tell God, our father, his daughter is here."

So, let me be the first to tell you, there are no pearly gates and no St. Peter. I don't recall much about my passing but I was 101 years old at my death so I couldn't tell you what I'd had for breakfast most of the time!

Now, when you die, that part about your life flashing before your eyes, that's true! It seemed I was remembering every minute detail of my life in rapid, vivid flashes: a teacher's face, a brightly colored dress from childhood, a kiss, an argument, the view from my apartment in France, a tax return...I was zipping through my thoughts and memories at what seems to be a blistering speed, when the atmosphere changed (I really can't describe it any other way) and I sensed a voice. It's a rich, sweet, smooth voice, like warm chocolate pudding. It said, "You asked to see me?"

I played it cool, "Maybe," I said and then just to be sure, I timidity go, "Are you God? And if so, where are you?"

And the voice says, "Yes. And I am everywhere all at once. I know you expected me to have a human body, but I don't. Never did."

From that moment on, I was in slack-jawed, thigh-smacking, hoot and hollering awe of God! The power washed over me like a tsunami of comfort and joy. It took the *"me"* out of me, leaving what I can only describe as a pure spirit, filled to the brim with questions.

In a flash, I completely forgot that I was chewing the fat with the Almighty and found myself pointing out that, in the Bible, it says we humans are created in God's image. How can God not have a body? I was too polite to say this out loud but God, picked up on it anyway.

"I understand your confusion and it was all a misunderstanding, sort of a typo," God said. "I told Moses that I made humans in my *imagination*...not in my image!

"You know," God continued, "most of what you call the Bible wasn't written by the people whose names appear on the books. Moses, Ezekiel, Jeremiah, Samuel, etc., they all started their books, but a lot of tinkering went on with them over the years. I cannot even begin to tell you how badly the rewrites botched circumcision! I mean, if someone told you right now that to be a good Jewish boy, you need to let a someone clip off your foreskin, wouldn't you say, "Ah, could you repeat that?"

"But I thought you were infallible," I said to God.

"I AM," God laughed. "Technically, if I do it, it isn't a mistake but, in this case, Abraham misunderstood about the foreskin thing, hence the mistake was his, not mine. Humans are fallible. Years later, I had Paul explain it in the book of Romans, but it was too late and to this day, little Jewish boys are still getting nipped."

I am beginning to think God would make a good lawyer but then I heard a hint of wistfulness creep into his voice. "But, in hindsight," God said, "there are things I would do differently. Menstruation was a terrible idea. So was anger. I never get angry! That whole 'wrath of God' thing is a human invention.

"I gave you guys anger just so you could blow off steam and fully appreciate love and contentment. You've never learned to appreciate love but y'all find all sorts of justification to hold onto some anger in all its forms: hate, revenge, ridicule, sarcasm, spite. Turns out, as your emotions and your hormones evolved, some of you chose the endocrine cocktail of hate over love every time. I did not see that coming. In retrospect, maybe not so good."

I had so many questions! And the first one was, "Can you take a form so I can see you?"

There immediately appeared a small, white pit-bull terrier mix with black spots and a short tail, wagging. Instantly, I recognized the dog as Paperclip, my son's childhood pet. Sorry about the moniker but that's what happens when you let your 3 yr. old name the dog!

"God, why on Earth did you decide to show up as Paperclip?"

"Well, first we are nowhere near Earth and secondly, you were thinking about him right before you died."

This was true. I had a picture of my son when he was 7, with the dog, on my nightstand. As the life left my body, I was wondering if I would ever see either of them again.

God knew exactly what I was thinking. Now, in Paperclip's image, God said, "your son and everyone you have ever known are here, but not in a way you can imagine just yet," and he continued, "Tell you what: You settle in and collect your thoughts. We'll chat again. No pressure. You can ask me anything, as much as you want, whenever you want. After all, we have eternity, right?"

"And what exactly does that mean," I asked.

God paused, then said, "Your body is gone. Your existence is no longer an act of perception, punctuated by your sense of time, movement, breaths and heartbeats. Your human existence and future have evaporated. All that is left is now. And now, is eternity."

And with that, Paperclip did a downward facing dog, followed by an up-dog with a yawn, and trotted off into oblivion. In his wake, he left what I can only describe as the crisp feeling of deeply inhaled fresh mountain air.

I was, however, no longer inhaling and there was no air or mountain involved. I felt new and light. I was radiant, full of hope, promise and infinite possibilities. I had just had a chitchat with a god who resembles a mutt dog and He had promised to come back for more!

So far, death was wonderful!

5

I'd been dead for a while when he arrived. At first, he thought I was just sleeping, but when he bent down to kiss my forehead, his lips were met with a stony cold flesh that made him recoil. He immediately rang for the floor attendant but knew it was too late. Within minutes of his arrival, the RN on duty came and, finding no pulse, called the EMTs to pronounce me dead.

The room was exactly as it had been for the past 11 years: neat and with the faint smell of gardenia. It was amply furnished with a white leather recliner and love seat, a coffee table, a floor lamp, two end tables on either side of the queen-sized bed, each sporting a matching Tiffany lamp.

On either side of the sliding glass doors that led to the courtyard, he had installed a pair of bookcases, floor to ceiling, for the 400 books I'd insisted on bringing to the nursing home. As he looked around the bright, sunny room, he stared at my body as if he believed I just might yet sit up at any moment and ask for a cup of coffee.

"Hello. Sorry for your loss." The condolences came from my friend, Nancy, a gnome-sized woman, tightly grasping a walker and standing just outside the doorway to the inner hall. Her white hair was expertly pulled back into a chignon and in the way of makeup, she wore only a little lipstick that complimented her smile. She was dressed in a simple navy-blue cotton shirt dress, the collar stylishly popped at the back of the neck, a strand of pearls and white sandals.

"She was a good friend. A good talker and a good listener," the walker-lady said. "I'm Nancy. We were friends."

"I'm Jake, her son," said the old man. He was holding a silver picture frame he'd just picked up from the bedside table. "Can you believe that's me?" He tilted the frame toward the old woman and pointed to the boy in the photo, standing next to a spotted dog.

"It was taken about 70 years ago. That dog had a good life! Lived to be 16…that's what, about 90 in human years? Not as long as Mom," he said with a sigh. "I am going to miss her."

"Well, me too, but I'll be talking to her soon enough, I suppose." said the old lady with a weak chuckle. Jake must have assumed she meant death was just around the corner for her as well. "In fact," the old lady said, "I'm going to go check on her right now." And with that, she pivoted on her walker and scooted away with surprising vigor.

Jake looked back at my shrouded body, "Sounds like you're going to have company," he said.

Jake started looking through my books, as if searching for something. When his hand fell on my old Bible, I couldn't help but smile. I guess he felt he should say a prayer or something, so he took out that ratty old Bible of mine, a hopelessly worn out, red leather-bound volume I had received from the county upon high school graduation. Yes, in 1939, rural southern counties often gave a Bible to each new graduating high school senior. It was even embossed with my maiden name.

He found it under H, not B (Holy Bible) and he smiled. I had shelved it in the fiction section, not with the reference books.

"Faith with reason," he said aloud, quoting one of my favorite sayings.

As he opened the pages to Psalms 23, a small envelope, the size of a thank-you note fell out. It was addressed to him.

Dear Jake,

Thank you for looking up the 23rd Psalm. So, that means I'm dead. Glad you still seek comfort and wisdom from the 'good book'.

Please know that I died unafraid and ready to go. At my age, you start to get curious about what happens when your body finally gives out. Whatever it is, I'm sure it will be ok, so don't worry about me, little one. I died looking forward to meeting my God and have no doubt it will be…unimaginable.

You'll find the original of my Last Will and Testament in the lower right dresser drawer. I outlived a husband and two wives. Whatever's left is yours and it's all in order, so shouldn't be any legal bullshit for you to deal with. Just take what you want and give the rest to the folks at the Goodwill store. I like the idea of leaving a little 'goodwill' on earth.

Don't forget, my cremation is already paid for. It's all explained in the Will. You can keep me in an urn or scatter me in the marsh near my last condo. I will leave that up to you.

We'll, that's about it. At your age, you're finally an orphan! I love you, little one, and I hope to see you again in Heaven, or whatever lies ahead."

Ma

By this time, you might be wondering how I've managed to communicate my story about being dead to you, the living. It's a long and convoluted tale that didn't begin with Kurt Vonnegut, but you must understand the Kurt Vonnegut connection, and a lot more about my friend, Nancy, so that's where I'll start.

A long time ago, Kurt Vonnegut wrote a book called *Slapstick*. In it, he referred to life after death as "the turkey farm" and described it as the most boring place ever. Clever, but total malarkey!

However, Vonnegut was onto something! His main character happens upon a pipe-like devise, (for reasons I will explain shortly, Vonnegut called it the "Hooligan") a mechanism through which he was able to communicate with his dead sister.

Now, my old friend, Nancy at the nursing home, had been visiting the dead for *years* but nobody believed her! Turns out, she had a fucking Hooligan!

Not long after my death, Nancy and I talked for what must have been years in her time but barely an instant for me. Anyway, she...Nancy, wrote it all down and ultimately got the damn thing published! And not just our conversations! She had tons of them!

Currently, she is living off the proceeds of the book, spending the last of her dotty days being interviewed on white Wicca podcasts and eating buckets of her favorite butter pecan ice cream.

Now, back to my budding relationship with God.

Questions for God...Why did I never think to make this list when I was alive? I mean, I was a Christian from the get-go, christened as an infant and confirmed at age 7. I was "born again" at 15 and never looked back. True, my image of God, my understanding of God evolved throughout my life, and I have never doubted the existence of a higher power.

As a child, I would say my prayers each night:

'Now I lay me down to sleep,
I pray the Lord my soul to keep.
If I should die before I wake, I pray the

Lord my soul to take.'

Some may find this prayer a bit morbid, conjuring the image of a child, fearing imminent death before morning. To my way of thinking, this simply meant God was there, ready to scoop me up in case I croaked before dawn. I found that quite comforting.

Back then, I vaguely imagined God as a kindly old man with a flowing white beard, sitting on a cloud-like throne, watching my every move. This version was quite popular in Sunday School and most Bible storybooks. Later, I came to think of God as less of a person and more of a 'presence,' existing 'somewhere'.

As it turned out, it doesn't really matter how you see and understand God. The fact that we can imagine God at all is the point: we were created in God's imagination, therefore our own imaginations are part of the universe and by extension, of God.

To everyone reading this, please start *now* to firm up your understanding of God. Also, it would be a good idea to prep for your interview with God! You'll thank me when you're dead!

At first, my recently human soul was still full of random questions like, aliens in the universe and what an epiglottis is for, but these notions melted away and my introspection became more focused:

11

Questions for God:

-What are your pronouns? (It had become a very trendy question to ask. But in my case, I wasn't nosing around for God's gender identity. I simply figured, if we are going to have a conversation, I needed to know).

-Do you take sides?

-Is Hell for real?

-Does love really conquer hate?

-Why does evil exist?

-Are evil and sin the same thing?

-Are souls recycled?

-Is there an end to all time?

-Did you knock-up Mary?

-Why did Jesus have to die?

-Why did you make races?

-Do you hate homosexuals?

-Are ghost real?

-Do animals have souls and are they here in heaven? And if so, can I get all my old pets back together again at the same time?

-Who are you, really?

But, before I forget, let me tell you about Heaven. It's not so much a place. It's more of a state of being (making air quotes here). There are no clouds, harps, robes, wings or streets of gold. No mansions in the sky, no bejeweled thrones. So far, I have not met any dead relatives or long-dead beloved pets. (Except God costumed as Paperclip). I have not been showered with virgins and there was no milk and/or honey. I have neither had to answer for my sins, nor have I been rewarded for good behavior.

I just *am*. Whatever it was that used to go on between my ears is all that's left. Call it my mind, consciousness, soul, spirit or all the above.

This state of just being can best be described by what it-is-not rather than what it is. It is an absence of everything negative. I feel no guilt, no shame. There is not the slightest inkling of anguish, pain, fear, anticipation or anxiety. Regrets, envy, malice, anger, jealousy, depression, revenge? Zip, zero, nil, null, void, bupkis.

What I am feeling is exhilaration and peace, all at once. It's that 'peace that passeth all understanding' thing. I am not looking forward to my next audience with God because I know God's already here! It would seem that time and space are meaningless.

And with that thought, the chocolate-warm-pudding-voice of good-ole Paperclip was back, asking me to have a go at my list of questions.

"How'd you know I was ready to talk?"

"A-, I'm God and B-, I am always listening. I know every prayer you've ever prayed, every thought you've ever had."

"Why didn't you answer my prayers then?" To which God guffawed and replied, "Oh, honey, I answered every one of them! It just wasn't always in ways you could perceive.

"Like most people, you did a lot of praying but you were too impatient and shallow to really pay attention to the answers! Most of the time, you prayed as if you were going to a vending machine to get a candy bar. Money in, candy delivered. Prayer in, answer delivered. It doesn't work that way."

I was about to ask God for an example when Paperclip said, "For example, you were 21 yrs. old, and you got drunk on White Russians and started throwing up all over your boyfriend's apartment. You begged me to let you die. Well, I did let you die, just 80 years later. But you have more questions, so shoot."

"Ok, let's get the existential stuff out of the way first. What exactly am I right now?"

"Well, you're dead. The body you thought of as you, is gone. Humans are completely recyclable! Y'all are supposed to die, and your bodies become worm food. Then, you guys started making up all kinds of rituals, embalming and cremating your leftovers. It was not supposed to be that

14

way. You see, *everything* is designed to be recycled. What you call your soul is just that part of me tucked into every living thing. Humans, all animals, plants, fungi, bacteria and viruses all have a little bit o' God in them and, when their physical form goes tits up, that God-bit comes right back to me."

"So right now, you are talking to yourself, and I am talking to myself?"

"We could not have put it more succinctly!" God said. "Every time you prayed, you were talking to yourself *and* Me. It's why prayer seems so intimate. Of course, intimacy creates risk and vulnerability. All that poetic stuff about knowing yourself and, to thine own self be true is essential to a good prayer life. It's how you get to know yourself and ultimately Me."

I was stuck in the "risk of intimacy" phrase. I had never even considered God feeling the risk of intimacy but since I was God and plants are God, viruses are God and all animals are God, it now made perfect sense. God really was everywhere! God felt and understood everything.

"All that time Mohamed was explaining the 'one' God, he was trying to say *we* are one *with* God. Moses with the burning bush? That was a metaphor for an energy that is never consumed. Remember the great I AM? I am, you are, we are and it's eternal. Now that's a conjugation for understanding the universe, uh?"

15

"So, tell us, God, where did we come from?"

"I have no idea," God said with a shrug and a sigh. "It all started with light. And the light contained whatever I Am." Here, He paused to think, presumably of a way He could explain the beginning of the universe so I could understand. "It was like a cosmic jigsaw puzzle," He continued, "with an infinite number of pieces. I started putting the pieces together (first, light pieces then dark pieces) and then, the pieces started putting *themselves* together! Protons, neutrons and electrons started forming atoms. Atoms started splitting and producing energy. There was banging and flashing, and the jigsaw puzzle just kept on getting bigger. To this very second, it is forming and keeps forming on and on and on. I have yet to see a corner or edge piece. There's just no end in sight."

"So, no Adam and Eve," I said with what must have seemed like disappointment.

"No, at least not as humans. Remember, you were made in my imagination, not my image. No beginning, no end. I *never* implied that man was first, and woman was second. Humans cranked that myth and perpetuated it to the detriment of half your species for thousands of generations.

"The same with races. I didn't create different races! You humans came up with the idea of sorting yourselves by skin tones. The very idea of superiority within your species based on skin color is absurd! How could anyone think the shade of a person's epidermis would have *anything* to do with his or her value? You might as well have sorted yourselves by the size of your uvulas!"

"What?" I said with genuine confusion.

"Uvulas," God repeated, "that fleshy bit that hangs in the back of your throat."

"Oh, that was originally on my list. I thought that thing was called an epiglottis."

"Nope, that would be the flap that keeps stuff from going down your windpipe when you swallow," God replied.

"Now the uvula, it mostly keeps food and water from going up your nose. Humans are the only animals that have one," God said but then raised his right paw, as if to check that thought.

"Although to be fully accurate, there are a few apes that have little uvulas, but you humans have the full ones."

"Ok. Uvula hangs on the back of my throat, epiglottis covers my trachea when I swallow…or used to," I replied. "And while we are on the subject of anatomy, why did you make the vulva and the uvula so similar in spelling but so different in purpose?"

"I didn't name the body parts! Humans did! Besides, that only happens in languages with Latin roots," God said

17

patiently. "The point is the arbitrary differences humans use to stratify themselves are just that: arbitrary.

"And don't get me started on the imaginary lines y'all draw, pretending parts of the earth belong to you! Walls, borders, gates, moats are all human ideas. Think you might lay claim to the moon and other planets? Guess what: They don't belong to you!" God rolled over on his back, stretching his legs in the air.

"I am fascinated by your creativity, arrogance and capacity for learning," God continued, "but you seem to require a lot of selfishness before you recognize the divisions you've hardened and the sadness they bring. Fortunately, these things have a way of evolving. Remember, the human concept of time means nothing to us."

"And us is...?" I said with great anticipation.

"Us is you, me, every living particle of matter and energy. You wanted to ask me about pronouns? Strictly speaking, it's third person plural, all the way. You are no longer you, so technically, you are we and I am we but for purposes of our conversations and your conversations with Nancy, I can be He or She and you can be I or me. Does that make sense?"

"Ok, so you will be you or He and I will be me or she, except when we are talking about us, then it's we?"

"Now, that could be a very catchy Broadway lyric," God mused. "Why don't you just call me God and avoid the pronouns all together, hmm"?

"Ok, God. Tell me about good and evil."

Paperclip/God sat up and used one of his rear paws to scratch his ear. Then he laid down and quickly (in a matter of sentences, really) explained good and evil.

"First off, you need to understand the two are not mutually exclusive. It is not as easy as saying Mother Teresa was good and Charlie Manson was evil. Think of good and evil as being interchangeable, depending on your perspective.

"For example, say you are starving, and you steal a loaf of bread. If you don't get caught, you think, 'that's good' and you fill your tummy. Intellectually, however you know stealing is evil. It was a bad thing to do to the owner of the bread. Someone tries to stab you. That is evil. You defend yourself and stab the attacker. Is that evil or good? It all depends on how you look at it."

"So, are you saying good, and evil are situational?"

"No, but without a moral compass, it can seem that way. Hewing closely to the Ten Commandment would go a long way toward eschewing evil. And of course, there is the Golden Rule. Humans can't completely avoid evil but if they work earnestly at treating others the way they want to be treated, they can do infinite good."

"And the good people go to Heaven?" I said as a tentative question.

"Nope," said God with a wink. "Y'all make your own Heaven and Hell right on earth. When you die, your pure and beautiful soul comes right back to me, whether you're Mother Teresa or Charlie Manson."

"And what if my soul is not so pure?" I said with some trepidation.

"You will experience this in graphic detail soon," God replied. "You see, 'hell' come from the Anglo-Saxon *hel*, meaning "hidden." The English root word for hell, *helan*, just means more specifically 'to hide the unsightly,' such as garbage, human waste, trash."

"This originally came from Aramaic, Jesus's language. It was written as *gehenna* or *gehenna dnoora* in Aramaic (that's what Jesus called it) and *sheol* in Hebrew. Both words, taken together meant the garbage dump. So," God continued, "when humans die, I literally take out the trash you've accumulated in your souls and I chuck it straight to *Gehenna Dnoora*! What remains is the spirit of Me in you, now coming back to Me. Understandably, the more garbage you have in your soul, the deeper it is embedded, the longer and more painful the extraction process becomes."

"So, we are basically good?" again, my statement was more of a question.

"Yes, most of what you'd call human nature tends toward goodness, kindness, helpfulness and empathy. Real evil is the deliberate intention to hurt others, to inflict pain, to kill for selfish, hateful goals. I didn't invent that. Humans did."

This was getting interesting!

"Nobody starts out evil," God went on," it takes a foothold when people are deprived of something. Could be food, water, money, love, freedom, equality, dignity. Wanting either makes people motivated or mean. Sometimes both. And when acquisition makes a person want even more, just for the sake of having more, the situation is ripe for sin."

Suddenly, I had an epiphany. "And deliberately evil motivation is sin, right?" I blurted out.

"You're getting the hang of this," God said as he rolled over on his side, all fours stretching in front of himself. "Deliberate evil is sin. That's why I am always sadly amused when humanity tries to attribute 'sin' to things like left handedness or homosexuality. Innate behaviors aren't sins. They just *are*. It's like saying a rock is sinful! It's just a rock for Christ's sake!"

"Oh, oh, let's talk about Christ! Did you really father a son and put him inside a virgin?"

"That's a very superficial explanation for what happened! It would have been a neat trick, but terribly unethical and it wasn't necessary. The whole virgin birth thing neither adds nor detracts from the importance of Emmanuel, the one you call Jesus Christ."

Paperclip/God stood up and shook then sat back down on his butt. His tail was wagging vigorously.

"Humanity was a mess. People waring, killing each other over land, enslaving and raping the captured, starvation and poverty for most just so a few could live as kings.

"Then, people somehow got the idea that instead of sacrificing each other to make Me happy, they could kill and burn animals, get this... *to the glory of God*!?" Incidentally, that's how barbecues got started! They made a big show of consecrating those burnt offerings but don't think for a minute all that good roasted goat, lamb and beef was going to waste!" God slid Paperclip's tongue across his lips.

"Anyway, the whole point of sending a Messiah was not a *quid pro quo* of me sacrificing my son and giving the rest of you a first-class ticket to eternal life! I thought I made that clear with the whole Abraham and Isaac episode. The point was, you are all the same no matter what, and just like Jesus, you are all worthy of eternal life. Jesus was less of a sacrificial lamb and more of a guide, a trail boss showing the way.

"It wounds me, the way you divvy yourselves up into camps. I've watched you do it by color, by gender, even by the imaginary tribes and countries you create. So, I sent Emanuel.

Deeply aware of My presence within him, Jesus watched. As he aged, he experienced the love of life, juxtaposed with your sometimes paralyzing fear of anything 'different'. He was scorned, mocked, ridiculed and laughed at. His story was that of the ultimate outsider, who for a brief moment, rode into Jerusalem like a rock star.

"When all his followers suddenly glimpsed the love and power of this young Jewish man on a donkey, you got scared. You saw him riding bravely among the waving palm fronds and realized He was about to change *everything*. If you were going to follow him, that meant you were going to have to give up your prejudices, your hate, your concepts of wealth and power. It was mass hysteria.

"So, in a spectacular display of groupthink, the mob coalesced around a plan to kill the messenger in the most ignominious way. Dying on the cross was the ultimate indignity, the ultimate shame. As a blood-thirsty mob, you clamored for his death, mistakenly assuming getting rid of

23

the messenger would make the realization of your selfish Godlessness simply go away."

God was right (duh!). I had been so giddy about the resurrection I'd glossed over what happened to put Jesus on the cross in the first place!

"So, you're saying" I ventured, "Jesus died for our sins, but especially for the sins of letting him suffer and be publicly humiliated, just so we could keep our hate and prejudices alive?"

God's tail was no longer wagging. He had closed his eyes and laid his lower jaw across his front paws. And in a flood of understanding, I blurted out, "And when you resurrected Him, that was like a big middle finger to the hubris of humanity!?" God, eyes still closed, He sighed.

What I took away from all this is: We're born the same, we die the same and in between, we need to love and help each other. People with selfish intentions, driven by fear, will try to diminish you. Bad things happen to good people and vice-versa. Living will eventually consume your body, but nothing can break God's love for us, for our souls' connections to Him and the rest of the universe. Only God can separate us from our sinful baggage and, as the prayer goes, *'deliver us from evil.'*

God opened his eyes, stood and shook his head so forcefully, his ears flapped against his jaws.

"Don't forget," He whispered, "Jesus went from hero to zero in the space of a week! He was no more divine than you! But his message came straight from me: 'Come to me, all who are weary and burdened, and I will give you rest'. The one thing Matthew got right!"

God and I thought about that for a while. It was especially clear to me now that if God could take the abused and broken Jesus from the cross and restore him, not only to life but to *eternal* life, he could surely restore me! Then, He spoke again.

"So, here's the skinny on the virgin birth thing: The Hebrew was mistranslated into Greek. Isaiah, in Hebrew wrote that the messiah would be born to a young woman. That's exactly what I told him, but in your New Testament, 'young woman' was translated into 'virgin,' hence, the so-called virgin birth. Jesus was born just like everyone else, but I inhabited His body, just to get a sense of what you humans were going through and let me tell you, it was an eye-popper!" He went on to explain that, while the Qur'an also gives a whole chapter over to Mary and the virgin birth, it doesn't make Jesus into anything more than a prophet. "The point was, God is in everything and everything is in God, and in the end, we are all One," God said.

"And that eye-popping bit...could you elaborate?"

25

"Oh, just your brains, hormones, your emotions, your interactions with others and your environment: It's a lot to juggle. The concepts of time and space, relationships, of living, loving and dying are so complicated, you can hardly take it all in. It's why I dished out what you call the Holy Spirit or the Holy Ghost. Boo!" God laughed.

"Hold the phone," I shouted. "Go back to the Holy Spirit! There's you, Jesus and this Spirit. That part I am familiar with, but you're saying you invented the Trinity just to comfort us?"

"I did," God replied. "Jesus was God in man, made manifest and as God, well, I am completely unfathomable, so I carved out a middle ground of this spirit of peace, faith, gratitude and compassion. The Buddhist have been tapping into it for centuries. The Dalai Lama and many other people have been very successful at living in the Spirit," God mused.

"Think of it as a river that some people are just canoeing down. They've sussed out all the emotional judgements and manufactured biases and left them on the riverbank. They know their bodies are temporary and fragile. They just try to live in this spirit-river, trusting it will take them where they need to be."

God crossed his front paws and laid his head on his front legs again and we silently meditated on the river of Spirit and its gentle currents.

A little more on the aforementioned Hooligan.

It was discovered by an elementary school janitor, named Sean Hooligan, who found that his mop bucket, when put into proximity to a length of pipe in his utility closet, set up a direct line of communication to the newly dead. When the Hooligan "rings" it doesn't really make a sound. Somehow, I just know when I can reach out to Nancy and at other times, it's Nancy, reaching out to me.

"How's tricks in the afterlife?" At 98, Nancy was somewhat basic in her conversation skills. She also tended to yell a little when speaking into the Hooligan.

The Hooligan starts out very clear but toward the end of our conversations, the audio quality begins to suffer and sounds like a flock of turkeys in the background. Hence, Vonnegut's reference to the afterlife as 'the boring turkey farm.'

"Well," I responded, "I have been chatting with God and so far, I have learned we are all God, Mary maybe wasn't a virgin (but it doesn't matter) and even God doesn't know how the universe started and when it all ends," I explained.

Nancy said, "Just as I expected. I bet you didn't meet your dead relatives or your dead pets either, did ya?"

Nancy had been talking to the newly dead for years, so she knew a lot about the afterlife.

"Did God take a specific form to greet you?"

"Old pet, actually," I replied. "My son's dog, Paperclip."

"That's a new one!" Nancy snorted. "When my wife, Bertie died, God showed up as Milton Supman, better known in this life as Soupy Sales! I could barely talk to Bertie; she was laughing so hard at all the things God/Soupy was dishing out."

The 'turkey noise' was starting up in the background so I knew my conversation with Nancy would soon be impossible.

"Say, Nan, how the hell did you wind up with the Hooligan? How did you know how to use it?"

"Well, my late wife, Alberta (everybody called her Bertie) was a primary school principal. When her janitor discovered he could hear voices through the pipe in the utility closet, he told Bertie. Neither of them thought too much about it. Thought it was a rogue AM radio signal, until one of the voices called Sean by name! Poor Mr. Hooligan thought he was going crazy!

"The voice, however, was a kid from the school who'd recently died in a hunting accident. He just wanted to tell Sean and Bertie it was he who had backed up the toilet in the boys' bathroom by flushing a bull frog. Seems another kid had been wrongfully punished for it and his little-boy soul wanted to make amends, both to the wrongfully punished and to the bullfrog. Seems, in his case, confession was good for his little soul because they never heard from the kid again.

"After that, whenever an acquaintance died, the two of them would settle Sean's mop bucket in the right place and talk into the pipe. Most of the time, it was a brief chat, nothing special."

"Well, when Sean died, Bertie told me about the voices and let me listen in. We started referring to the mop bucket and the pipe as 'The Hooligan.' Alberta loved the author, Kurt Vonnegut and wrote him a letter about the Hooligan, thinking it would make a great plot line for a book. We called it 'Heaven and the Hooligan'. She got a nice form letter back from Mr. Vonnegut but nothing specific. Then, out comes Slapstick and the rest, as they say, is history.

"I sat in on a few calls before ole Bertie died and when I asked the school to give me the bucket and the pipe, they did...no questions asked.

"Now, I have the Hooligan set up in my clothes closet at the nursing home. Seems all I need do is call out a name of someone freshly departed and y'all pick up!"

And that was how Nancy added my story to her collection of Hooligan case studies. The book she wrote never made the best seller list, but it does still have a solid eBook following and everyone who's read it and died seems to contact Nancy. It reached the point that she had to use an Excel spreadsheet just to schedule the calls!

Nancy did tell me that she was never able to initiate a conversation with anyone historically famous, like Joan d'Arc, or anyone for that matter, who had been dead for more than an hour or two. In short, we're thinking ghost don't exist or they're just remarkably good at concealment.

Nancy did, however, talk briefly with Farrah Fawcett, Ed McMahon and Michael Jackson by way of Cecil Willis. Cecil was a resident of the nursing home who passed away on the same day as Michael, Ed and Farrah. Cecil said Michael was devastated at the way Ed's and Farrah's passing were ignored by the media compared to his…for a hot minute. Ed and Farrah didn't give a 'flying rat's ass,' as Ed put it. Within a moment after contacting Nancy, they all four happily melted into the energy of God, never to be heard from again.

When God returned, I could tell something had changed. Paperclip seemed larger than he was in life, as if he'd bulked up on steroids. Then, I realized, perhaps it was I who had gotten smaller! I can't really explain it because I no longer had a body, so size wasn't even a thing. It was simply my perception of "me" that had dwindled.

"Any more questions," He asked?

"Just one. Could you elaborate on how we were formed in your imagination?"

"Oh that!" God seemed elated by the question. The air around us softened, became tinted, then electrified, as if lightning bolts were shooting from pastel, cotton candy.

"The easiest way to explain it is:

I created you.

Part of Me is in you.

This includes your imagination.

Therefore, your imagination is part of me.

It's a subtle thing, how I live in humans and in your imaginations. I am by no means imaginary, yet every prayer, every conversation we have begins between your ears.

Your neuroscientists have nibbled around the edges of this, sometimes calling it the "right brain." That's about as accurate as saying, 'the ocean is wet'. It's true but that's a very simplistic description of something as vast and life-giving as earth's oceans."

"So, you're saying imagination is more than just right-brain creativity," I ventured.

"Oh, yeah!" God replied. "Beaucoup more. There's what y'all call the prefrontal cortex and temporal lobe along with communication centers and the various outer and inner regions of the parietal cortex."

"So, my whole brain is my imagination?"

"Everything about you is your imagination! From the moment you're born, you're experiencing life. Every little encounter is hooked onto the infinite pegboard of memory as you do and see, touch, taste, hear. It's a mini version of my own experience with creating the universe. The pieces of information and experience flood in and arrange themselves in ideas and memories. Before long, these snapshots start to build and merge. You leap from making sounds to words. You make noise, then music. Colors become lavish, imaginary landscapes. What starts as an idea becomes a building, a symphony, a medical breakthrough, an act of kindness or anger, and yes, a prayer. When you give yourself over to imagination in prayer, you're able to tap into the universe of power and possibility that is what some have called the Mind of God."

Suddenly, the phrase, 'The communion of saints, the forgiveness of sins, the resurrection of the body and the life-everlasting' popped into my consciousness.

"Exactly," God whispered, and it felt as if he'd kissed my cheek.

"Ok," said God. "Before I suck you up into the energy of the Universe, the Universe wants you to know a few things. You need to just listen. I will give you a chance to ask questions but with what I have to say, most of your questions will be answered."

God's nostrils were about the size of manhole covers now, but that warm, chocolate voice was as smooth as ever. He took a deep breath and so he began:

32

"What you call space is not empty. It is in fact boiling with matter. As a human, you perceived reality through your senses but there was, is, so much you miss. The cells, the atoms, the protons, neutrons, electrons, quarks are all part of the fabric you cannot see, yet it's there, binding the universe together.

"I designed you to adapt to your environment. That's what you are doing now…your environment now is almost pure energy. There's still some negative energy, however, that you have generated within yourself. Jung called it the "shadow self" and it's all the negative self-talk, the fears you have internalized. These are the dark impulses and shame you have accumulated over a lifetime, however most of them were acquired when you were very young.

In an instant, your mind, consciousness, subconscious will slip into the ocean of life. The self that you were on earth is like a wave. It rose from the ocean. It grew and crested. Now, you are ebbing and flowing back into the ocean of pure spirit and energy.

"But before that, we need to shake loose those destructive bits you've manufactured about yourself. It's going to hurt. Think of it as the spiritual equivalent of having a hard scab ripped off."

The imagery of waves, shadows and scabs was coming toward me at a dizzying speed. With each spoken word,

God was gently lowering me into a slowly darkening abyss, alternately exploding with fire and ice.

"From the moment you were born, you have struggled to shape yourself as a unique and separate entity. Learning to walk, eat, regulate your body functions, communicate. These milestones of autonomy were praised as life skills and of course they're necessary for civilization. The side effects however often throw humans into an ever-devolving spiral of loneliness and isolation."

For the first time in my life and death, I felt what it was like to be separated from God.

What happened next was my master class in salvation. God spun me into a holy roll! Somewhere within me, I began to hear a faint melodic, harmonic oscillation, at once sinister and somehow, perfectly normal. It was a background complement to the voice of God, as He continued, "No one is born angry, anxious, depressed, hateful, fearful or greedy," he began. "You learned these feelings as you strived to become independent. And all the while, the peace and confidence you were seeking was inside the community and vulnerability you feared.

"To join the energy of the universe, you'll have to revisit some of the worst days of your life and see how much easier they could have been if only you had opened yourself to the help of the energy that was always there to support you."

After a long pause, I whispered, "Instead, I wallowed in self-pity. I got drunk on my autonomy and denied You, didn't I?"

"Yeah. A lot of you find power, drugs or booze or some other form of denial." God replied. "You all think you're the only one who feels that way."

At this point, Paperclip had become so big, he'd vanish or, I had become so small, I'd vanished. (Does it really matter which)?

God continued, "This next part may seem like punishment or an exorcism but it's just a purge, a spiritual up-chuck, of all the residual evil and pain you're still holding. So, baby, we are now going to rock your soul in the bosom of Abraham!"

The atmosphere began to pulsate to the music in a visually harmonious language, not of words but of clear, sharp and vivid imagery, much like the images I 'felt' upon dying but this time, I could understand what I was meant to see.

A spanking for drawing in crayon on my closet wall when I was 2 years old. Injustice. (*You did nothing wrong!*)

Laughed at for having dirty ankles in first grade. Humiliation (*You did nothing wrong!*)

You talk too much. You stole money for candy because all the other kids had allowances and you didn't. You had nightmares. You were spanked for crying!? You made up wild stories to get attention. You accidentally started a brush fire in the backyard. You shot your sister's friend in the face with a rubber band. You brought home stray dogs. You were never good at anything, you drank too much, never wanted, never loved, queer, stupid, a terrible parent, narcissistic, anxious, depressed, alcoholic, the butt of all jokes, lazy, unworthy gullible fool, a big fat lie of a life.

You said yes, yes, yes when you wanted to say no. Everybody's doormat. Never worthy, a dismal failure. Not your fault and none of it was true!

The disgrace and ignominy I had invented for myself exited my being. Like sharp knives, shards of glass and razor blades, the pain of a lifetime sliced through my soul and emerged as brilliantly hued butterflies and flowers. As the pulsing-humming subsided, all the selfish, egotistical angst and pain I had greedily clung to for 101 years died with a "poof".

"What the fuck just happened," was my only thought.

"Oh, that was me taking out the trash," God sighed. "It is always the same, yet it never gets old. All the horrors you have suffered, all the lies you told yourself about yourself, gone. We just roto-rooted your soul, converting all that negative baggage you've been carrying around into positive energy and the breath of life."

Whose life?" I wondered.

36

"Just plain old, miraculous life," God said. "From crabs on the beach to grass in the jungle, elephants, mice and humans...the spark of life that animates it all."

By now, Paperclip was gone and only the exquisite voice of God remained. Yet, it was no longer outside of me! When God spoke, it was as if I were talking to myself, as if I knew the questions and the answers all at the same instant. There was no more duality. No more good/bad, right/wrong, up/down, black/white. Everything just...is.

"Now what?" I asked. "Reincarnation?"

"Noooooo..." God's voice was barely audible. It sounded like deep, tubular wind chimes.

"You're done. Remember? Now is eternity. Now, you will flash as lightening, roar as thunder. You will fall with snow and melt into streams, lakes, rivers and oceans. Your ideas, compassion, empathy and understanding will drift into the hearts and minds of the living, and they will think, invent, create, destroy and rebuild."

My journey, in this fresh life, pure of spirit with God, unfolded as delight, enthusiasm, contentment, tranquility, peace, ardency, faith, empathy for others: The peace that passes all understanding.

Living mortals will continue to struggle in the duality of flesh and I have a front row seat. Yet, their messy bodies, their swings from ego to altruism, their pain and bliss, their day and night are none of my concern.

37

"He will wipe away every tear from their eyes, and death shall be no more, neither shall there be mourning, nor crying, nor pain anymore, for the former things have passed away," God thought.

"Remember when you were baptized? You were, 'sealed by the Holy Spirit and marked as Christ's own forever'? Well, getting sprinkled with a little water had nothing to do with it!" God thought.

"You have always been you *and* part of Me, the energy of the universe. The 'Holy Communion' is what you are experiencing now! It just means sharing, tapping into the power that was always within you and within your reach."

"Like Dorothy and the Ruby Slippers," I thought dreamily with a little chuckle.

"Oh, I love that simile! You were Dorothy, moving through life into heartless, mindless, cowardly adventures, until you discovered *you* were searching for Me, for the universal wellspring of…

"Peace and home," I whispered, completing the thought. "The peace that passes all understanding."

"Yeah. Peace, my love," mused God.

And the last thing I clearly remembered was the momentary urge to say, in a Porky Pig voice, "Th-th-th-that's all folks!" Instead, I joined the universe in uttering a soft, rolling, thunderous, harmonically chanted, "Namaste."

Note from Nancy:

The preceding text was rendered by yours truly. I can't promise it's true, but it's what Betty told me.

Who can say? If God gave us our imaginations and if imagining God helps us understand ourselves AND God, well, is that so hard to believe? I mean, humans have always invented outlandish propositions to explain our existence, make sense of our actions and hypothesize about the afterlife.

No one faith or religion has a lock on spirituality! In fact, religions have been responsible for most of the wars and prejudices we humans ascribe to. A little less emphasis on our differences and a little more acceptance of what makes us alike would be nice.

We share the fear, loneliness and self-doubt, as well as the love, joy and enthusiasm that mark the milestones of our earthly existence. Druids, Hindus, Muslims, Jews, Christians, Buddhist, the agnostic and the atheist all share the human story, with every breath and beating heart.

When the last chapter is written and the book of life closes, I find it infinitely joyful to believe I will be winnowed from the sins I have committed, the sadness and the fear accumulated in life, and returned to the pure, heavenly energy whence I came. My experience with the Hooligan has left me optimistic about my death, whenever it may come, and I am not afraid.

What follows are some of my favorite encounters with the Hooligan. They just go to show that life after death is as unique to every human being as our very fingerprints.

I hope you enjoy reading them (the stories, not the fingerprints) as much as I enjoyed hearing them and faithfully recording ever single word.

Gavin's Story

"Everyone dies, but no one is dead."

- Tibetan saying

Be yourself. Everyone else is already taken.

- Oscar Wilde

What just happened? I'm on my bike, flying down I-95, drafting on a tractor-trailer and WHAM, I am floating above that big rig, (now jackknifed) looking at the bloody mess that used to be my body! Am I dead? I don't want to be dead!

Those were the first thoughts that ran through...I guess, my mind? Hovering above the scene, I see the rig's

41

driver kick open the passenger-side door and squeezing himself out of the mangled, overturned cab. There's a deer carcass, flopping, in the median. The truck driver is gasping for breath between ragged whimpers of, "I'm ok, I'm ok, oh fuck, I'm ok". In the distance, the pastoral sound of birdsongs. Mist is rising with the sun.

The driver scrambles, hands and knees to the ground. He's scanning the empty interstate, but no vehicles are approaching. He sees the front wheel of my bike, still spinning, partially blocked from view by the overturned trailer. He stands up and staggers toward the back of the truck's trailer to get a better look. Good thing he did, too! Just about the time he reached my body, his cab exploded. He shrieked, hit the pavement and covered his head as a big boom and a swoosh of flame and black smoke shot up into the sky around me but I didn't feel a thing.

As the smoke cleared, everything got lighter. Like a watercolor painting, swirls of tinted light, blues, wisps of purple, white and pink began to dance around me in soft pastels. The colors began to define me, to outline a new body. And there I was. I must have had eyes because I could see my new, ephemeral hands and feet! A soft, comfortable chair appeared beside me. Instinctively, I sat down.

I must have had ears, too because a little snorting noise alerted me to the pastel tan deer that was nuzzling my right hand, as if looking for some attention.

"What the f-?" I mumbled and instantly I hear a giggly little girl voice say, "It's a deer, silly!"

This new information came from the pastel clouds in front of me. There emerged a being wearing what appeared to be wildflowers around its head and wrists and ankles. It had a radiant white smile and dark brown eyes, but the rest of the body looked like shimmering swirls of cotton candy that quickly coalesced into a perfect little person who was all at once familiar and other worldly.

"I bet you never saw a deer's spirit before," she said. "They're common here. They get hit by cars a lot. You got hit by a car, too, didn't 'cha?"

And before I could respond, she had jumped into my lap and was snuggling her little bald head under my chin. She smelled faintly of lavender.

"It was a truck," I said, "and to be clear, the truck hit the deer, then I hit the truck. It was a terrible mess!"

"No, it wasn't!" The little girl giggled. "It all happened exactly the way it was 'pose to. You may call it a 'mess' but it was the deer's time. It was your time. The truck driver? Not so much." She shrugged and patted my cheeks with her hands.

"So," I said with a sigh, "I'm dead, right?

43

"You surely are," she replied, nodding once, emphatically. "And the deer, too," she added as she hopped off my lap to hug the deer spirit.

"And you are?" I asked with absolutely no preconceived idea of what her answer might be. Oddly enough, I wasn't the least bit upset anymore about the prospect of being dead! That initial jolt of denial was gone. The only feeling I had was one of intense curiosity.

"Me? In Hebrew, I'm Malach. In French, they call me Ange. It's Inger in Romanian. The Chinese say Tian Shi. English speakers call me Angel."

"Ok, if you're an angel, what am I?"

"You're *you*, silly!" she said with a genuinely delightful laugh. "You're one of a kind, totally unique in the universe, never to be repeated!"

"And this is…what?" I said as I looked around.

"This is what some humans might call Heaven or the afterlife, but I know you don't believe in that. And all those years, you thought life-after-death was just a big hoax, invented by the world's religions. That's funny!"

I wasn't sure I believed her. I mean, I had spent my 26 years on earth just fine without a "smidgen of religion," I used to say. My parents taught me honesty, fairness, kindness. I had a morale code. I believed in truth and integrity. I treated people they way I wanted to be treated but there was no god pushing me to be good and certainly no devil tempting me to misbehave!

The stories told by the world's religions were inspiring I guessed, but certainly not true! Now, this angel (or maybe just Angel, or perhaps THE angel, I didn't know) was telling me my beliefs were…funny?

Angel continued petting the deer and, somewhat proudly said, "I'm what you might call your guardian angel. Every living thing on earth has one. This little deer is mine, too. It all comes down to" and Angel paused as if trying to remember something tricky, then said, "deoxyribonucleic acid! I'm part of his DNA," and she pointed to the deer, "just as I'm part of your DNA. See, you, that deer and I are still everything our DNA made us. We're just…what's the word…*virtual* now." She then poked her finger through my chest, and it responded like Jell-O. It moved, then snapped right back into place, exactly as I had seen a DNA double-helix behave in a 9th grade video! I saw it, yet I didn't feel a thing.

"What happened to my body? Where's my body now?" I said, and again, my question was without fear or trepidation.

"Good questions!" Angel whispered. I heard it but realized her lips had not moved. I tried thinking "Angel," and immediately I knew she was listening. My next thought was, "What?"

"This is how we converse," she "thought" to me. "You might call it telepathic but it's also empathetic, sympathetic and sometimes, psychedelic!" She punctuated this little recital with tap dance moves. "Some scientists call it 'epigenetic activity' or something that happens over and above what they fully understand about DNA.

"Your old body is still full of cells and genetic material, but without oxygen, it dies quickly. All the organic matter decays but the electrical activity from your mitochondrial DNA reforms a body of pure energy. Your DNA hasn't changed, but death has changed how your DNA performs. Its evolution from now on is purely spiritual.

"This spiritual DNA has always been there," Angel continued, "Its methylation to spiritual receptors is one epigenetic mechanism that changes the way your virtual genes perform. You haven't "gone" anywhere! You're simply now able to function as pure energy."

I just stared blankly, and Angel continued.

"As your consciousness expands, you're going to need more intellectual space. Speech, your senses, are just a few of the many human things you'll leave behind. You'll quickly forget your past life, to make room for all the new stuff your DNA will do."

"But I don't want to forget my life," I blurted out, jumping from my chair. "I want to remember the people I loved, the places I've been, ...*who I am*..."

Angel gently pushed me back, cooing, "sit, sit, sit". She held my shimmering hands and explained, "Do you remember being in the womb?" She asked.

"Of course not," I scoffed.

"And why do you suppose that is?" she asked.

"Well, for one thing, my fetal brain was mush!"

"Right," Angel said. "Now, imagine that almost everything your DNA did for you in this last life is just as unimportant now as your womb DNA was to your human life on earth. Zero, right?!

You are about to go from caterpillar to butterfly! Remembering how to be a caterpillar will not serve you. Sperm, egg, zygote, embryo, fetus, baby, adult, they're all just stages. You're just in transition to the next stage. Try to enjoy it."

And with that assignment, Angel's voice faded. Somewhere in my mind's eye, l saw an ambulance, lights flashing, headed toward my dead body and the burning truck.

The paramedics gently removed my cracked helmet. They lifted my twisted corpse onto the stretcher. They straighten my impossibly broken neck, covered my bloody body with a crisp white sheet and loaded it into the ambulance. I was touched by the reverence, the tenderness they displayed and though I couldn't feel their touch, I was overwhelmed by their deep sense of reverence for a life that was no more.

Another EMT was tending to the truck driver, who was still shaking, sobbing inconsolably. In jagged breaths, he would blurt out random words, "sorry" and "Jesus" and "why" were the most oft repeated. The EMT had his arm around the guy and just kept patting his shoulder, saying, "It's ok, you couldn't have known there was a biker back there. That deer was just trying to cross the road. It was an accident. You're going to be ok. Not your fault."

Gradually, I became aware of hundreds, maybe thousands of spirit bodies, just like Angel and me, floating above and swishing among the humans on the ground. They were simultaneously passing through the bodies of the humans and...dancing? It was like some cosmic Cirque du Soleil, but without trapezes.

They were moving through the humans, but also in and out of the truck, the deer carcass, the road, the grass, trees, even the soil. As the sun climbed, police and firefighters arrived. A large tow truck began winching up the overturned rig and more commuters began to pass. The spirits went through them, too. I asked Angel what was happening, and her response was instantaneous, even though she was nowhere in sight.

"This is what we do. Whenever there is a violent shift in the balance of life on earth, no matter how large or small, we rush in to heal the psychic trauma. When humans witness death and injury, you have a visceral reaction. Your hearts race, your senses sharpen, many of you pray. That's us, working through you." But then, she quickly added, "we're there for the good stuff, too! Most of what you call 'lucky' is us."

"And everyone who dies becomes a spirit?" I asked.

Angel thought for a moment and then slowly said, "Yes, but not every spirit is the same. You see, now that you're dead, I will no longer be your guardian. I'm going to move on, maybe to another dimension, maybe to guard more living things. I'll know when it happens."

"And me?"

"Oh, you're going to become his guardian!" and she indicated the truck driver. "He's a Christian and he really needs to know that your death wasn't his fault. You're going to help him with that, but you're not ready yet. Your newly dead consciousness is still like the fetus in the womb, not fully formed or informed."

And with that, I left the scene of my death, dissolved and reappeared, this time in what I recognized as my parent's kitchen. My mother, a schoolteacher, was enjoying her last cup of coffee as my dad, a construction foreman, shoved his wallet in his hip pocket, getting ready to head out the back door to work. Just as he kissed Mom goodbye, his cell phone rang. Dad, grimaced and said, "Jesus, I hope this isn't somebody calling in sick."

It was the South Carolina Highway Patrol, informing him of my death. His disbelief was the first thing I felt, followed by a slowly rising panic. At the same time, he was listening and asking questions. His mind was processing how to stay calm, so as not to upset my mother. Somehow, I understood it all.

Without any thought or preparation, my spirit went straight to my mom. I tried, without knowing how, to contain the spark of anxiety that was growing as she heard my father's questions: "When? Where was he? He was doing what!?" The spark burst into flame when she heard Dad say, "Are you sure it's him?"

The ensuing tornado of terror, grief and disbelief was so powerful, it kicked me hard, away from my mother's soul. Angel gently whispered, "It's always like this when people die unexpectedly," she said softly. "You can't help her yet."

With my parents now coming to terms with my demise, I was gently pulled away from my life on earth, reborn in my new reality, into a new dimension of unfathomable grace. Juxtaposed with my parents' anguish and grief, I felt so *lucky* to be dead!

All thoughts about my life on earth, my past, were gone. No trepidations, just an exhilarating sense of anticipation for what lay ahead. You know that feeling when you're about to start a great vacation? That's how it felt.

"Angel, what are we? Where are we? And why all the references to DNA? Earlier you said, 'this is what we do.' What'd you mean by that?"

Angel was hovering, just at my eye level, sometimes twisting into what looked like yoga poses, sometimes turning slow somersault in the air.

"This feels so good! You ought to try it," she said, lazily.

When I didn't move, she settled into a lotus position. It was only then that I realized neither of our bodies had genitals, no hair, no nails, just our well defined, cotton-candy-colored bodies of smoky pastel Jell-O.

This lack of private parts should have freaked me out, I mean, my dick was gone! Testicles too! Instead, I was amused and even said out loud, "Would you look at that?"

Angel looked, but quickly moved on, as if my unpacked package was of zero interest.

"Ok," Angel said, clapping her hands together. Then with the air of an official tour guide, she began, "Welcome to your next life. In the first one, you were a product of matter, biology and chemistry. You were formed in the womb and grew, two cells, four cells, millions of cells, all doing exactly what your DNA told them to do.

"Then, you hit your second life, out of your mom and into the physical world! You grew some more. You were nurtured and fed. You became a distinct individual. And, as an individual, you made the decision to go drafting on a tractor-trailer. It was all in your DNA.

"And now," Angel continued "you are in your third life, reborn to a new body, in a new dimension of reality. Just as your DNA dictated all your physical attributes, your spirit, your soul are also determined by your DNA. Isn't it perfect?" she asked with a shrug and the sweetest smile.

"The genetic energy within your ancestor's DNA, pulled you here," she held her arms out wide to illustrate the vast space we were in. "And the genetic energy, pulsing on earth, keeps us in touch with everything that lives there. Human philosophers and theologians have nibbled around the edges of this forever," Angel continued, rolling her eyes in mock weariness. "Aristotle and Thomas Aquinas each held the notion that there is a soul, unique to every living organism. This "soul" is the thing that gives an organism its character, as well as the essence of that species. Thus, plants were viewed as having a vegetative soul, animals a sensing soul, and humans an intellectual soul."

Angel's childlike voice continued. "Albert Einstein called this soul factor a 'mysterious action at a distance'. It has caused many scientists, including him, to question whether quantum physics is a complete or correct theory of 'reality' and how we experience it.

The non-local nature of the spiritual leads many people to believe that spiritual phenomena cannot be explained scientifically, but humans will eventually figure it out, just as you eventually understood the connection between sex, reproduction and gestation, between nature and nurture."

"So, what do we do now?" I asked.

"Oh, this is the best part!" Angel said as she hovered right in front of me. I was sitting, cross legged, still in the comfy chair when she slid her little hands beneath my knees and, with no effort at all, raised me up and showed me that I could hover, just like her.

"We are spirits, the electrical essence of our former flesh and blood. Our world is all around the earthly world and we understand all their languages in pure thought. We watch them. We look after their emotional needs. Mostly, we help them."

"How?" I asked.

"Oh, lots of ways! Like when you tried to console your mother. Her Angel will help her when she prays. Right now, she and your dad are still in denial. They're still hoping it's all a mistake. They're calling your phone, calling your friends, even though the patrolman told them it was you. Once they accept that you're dead, their angels will help them grieve."

And with that, we seem to meditate on sadness. I could sense Angel's thoughts as she led me through the many aspects of grief.

"Grief starts with an unbearable emptiness, defined by psychological anguish. It's the end of normal. It destroys the mental scaffolding we built for our future selves. Grief never leaves our souls. It has a half-life, always diminishing but never fully gone. Life goes on, yet we never completely forget our grief. It's a sidebar that changes us but should never be the main storyline."

Even as I understood this, I could feel all my own little griefs collapsing in on themselves, popping like soap bubbles. Where I was going, grief was an ever-diminishing memory.

Angel ended our meditation on grief by saying "We do lots of fun stuff, too," and she punctuated her remark with a backflip.

"Humans call us angels, poltergeists, demons, ghosts, apparitions, though we rarely…I mean *rarely* materialize.

"We are that feeling of comfort that comes over humans when they pray. But we are also the stuff of conscience. Humans really do have a little voice inside their heads, helping them weigh a dozen inputs and act in the blink of an eye," and then Angel whispered, "That's us!

"Part of it is, of course their own imaginations but our energy supplements theirs and it's just enough for them to feel it. It's all very subjective. Quantum phenomena and spiritual phenomena both depend on the observer, right? The act of observation can affect what is being observed or felt, so we try to stay out of sight."

As I was wishing I'd done better than a C-minus in high school physics, Angel continued. "It all comes down to information, stored as energy, in our DNA." Angel then stood erect and pointed one finger in the air, looking very professorial, she said, "As Einstein put it:

'Everything is energy and that's all there is to it. Match the frequency of the reality that you want, and you cannot help but get that reality. It can be no other way. This is not philosophy, this is physics.' You have experienced the reality of life," Angel said. "Now, your DNA has kicked into a new frequency and you're dialing up a whole new reality of pure energy. You can still interact with the old reality, but not as a living organism."

Changing the subject abruptly, Angel brightened up and asked, "Did you know that you no longer have internal organs? You don't ever need to eat ever again, yet you can instantly recall every great taste or sensation you've ever had." You don't have a crack in your ass anymore either," she said. Then, dropping her head between her knees, stuck her butt in the air to emphasize the point. I couldn't help but laugh. It was the purest feeling of joy I'd ever felt, and it was just a butt joke!

"That's the spirit!" She said and giggled at her pun.

For an indeterminate time, I practiced floating and flipping. It felt sort of like swimming but without water or the need to come up for air. Angel was there but she wasn't communicating, at least not with me. Every so often, a cotton-candy-like being would zip past us, as if off on an urgent mission.

"So, Angel," I said as we flipped and turned, "when do I become a guardian angel? When do I get to start looking after the truck driver?"

"Oh, you'll know. It usually starts with him or someone close to him, praying. You'll hear it. He'll ask things like, 'why me' and he'll think things like, 'I wish I'd died,' but you'll be there to help steer his thoughts into answers and you will help him re-scaffold his future. You'll also help him lighten up and become less selfish and more aware of his influence on the lives around him. I like to use humor for that."

"How do you mean?"

"Well, "and with a conspiratorial cut of the eyes, Angel said, "I do something totally unexpected!"

"Like what?" I asked. I was hoping for some real insight into how to be a DNA spirit, when Angel said, in complete seriousness, "Inappropriate laughter. Cause someone to snicker at a funeral! Make something funny happen at the most unexpected moment. One person tries to repress it, then another. Trying to suppress laughter, in the most inappropriate moments, is irresistible to humans. It shows them just how temporal their grief is, shows them they can still laugh, that there is still joy in the world. It works every time!"

"And just how do you do that?"

"Oh, a zillion ways!" Angel said. "Now, a fart noise is the most sure-fire way to get suppressed laughter, but for real artist, like us, there are more subtle and refined scenarios. Like, one time, during a summertime graveside service, I caused a breeze that blew the celebrant's robe over his head, revealing nothing but his brogans, black knee socks and a Speedo underneath! Another time, (and this was some of my best work) I had someone's phone go off in the middle of the funeral service," she said with a very smug look.

"We'll, that's not particularly funny," I said, not to be ugly, but just stating a fact.

"Yeah, but the ring tone was 'Another One Bites the Dust.' Just watching that pallbearer frantically fishing the phone out of his pocket while trying not to drop the casket was funny enough, but as soon as the widow recognized that riff, she and her two adult children could not hold it together! In seconds, the whole congregation lost it! It was rapturous! And, when the priest said, 'We've all heard of souls being called home to Jesus, but this is the first time I've heard the call come in on a cell phone, from Freddy Mercury, at the funeral!' The congregation loved it.

Then, there are what I called the scamp spirits. They do nice things, but they also do pranks. They make you forget your keys, mess up your flights, cause flat tires, just to see what you'll do. The scamps also decide who wins all games of chance! Did you ever win at roulette or blackjack? That was the scamps! Have you ever walked into a room and forgotten why you went there? That's them!"

"But, back to the DNA thing…," I said. "Am I really still uniquely me?"

"Absolutely!" said Angel. "You are one of a kind, but you are also about to become part of something much bigger and much more satisfying than an individual."

Before I could inquire further, Angel held up her palm, as if to preempt my questions.

"Remember, at the scene of your death, you saw all the spirits moving in and around every living organism? You thought then that the love and reverence you felt was coming from the EMTs and the police on the scene. Some of it was, but most of that was amplified by the spirits. You're going to become part of that. You will soon start communicating with all the spirits, not just me and you will hear and understand them all at once! It's like a giant pipe organ and every note is in perfect, exquisite harmony."

As Angel told me this, I did indeed begin to hear the low bass rumblings of that organ. I saw, somewhere in my mind, the swirling of uncountable pastel spirit-bodies. They were whipping up a tornado of ethereal sounds and colors. At the center of this stew of hues and sounds, I could feel my parents as they started to grieve my death.

They were sad beyond measure, sadder than they had ever been before and they were angry! Yet, I could already feel their future and I knew they would survive, with their faith and help from the spirits. This was a moment of epiphany, a realization not just of the power of prayer, but an immersion within the *energy* of prayer! This energy was as real as the rocks and trees. I'd just never, could never, understand it as a human.

My consciousness slowly shifted from the tornado of my parent's grief to the driver of the truck that killed me. He was in his home, with his wife and two kids. He was calmer than the last time I saw him, but still, I could feel an emptiness within him. It was as if all the promise of the future had been violently torn away. What remained was a gaping hole of fear and uncertainty, dark with regret and a longing to return to that split second before he hit the deer.

Instinctively, I went to that place and tried to fill the hole with forgiveness…not me forgiving him, but encouragement for him to forgive himself.

"Daddy?" His little girl said as she climbed into his lap. "Let's watch the Minions!" And with that, I planted an idea in the little girl's mind. She giggled, like the Minions sometimes do, made a raspberry noise, and minion-giggled again, poking a finger into her daddy's belly.

For the first time since the accident, my truck driver smiled, hugged his little girl and then chuckled softly while kissing the top of her head. His eyes teared up. It was her future that danced across his thoughts and for an instant, he could vaguely see himself through her eyes. In that moment, he forgot about the traumatic events of the morning, and he was Daddy again, her one and only Daddy.

As a spirit, I quickly understood that it wasn't my uniqueness that allowed me to commune with this stranger, my killer. It was our similarities! In fact, my DNA was communicating with the DNA of every living thing surrounding me!

Even though we are unique, we share 99.9% of our DNA. Genetically we are virtually the same. Heck, 80% of my DNA was the same as Angel's deer and 41% of my DNA can also be found it a banana! What makes us uniquely different also makes us alike. Is it any wonder then that we are all so much more alike than we are different?

The truck driver didn't know why, but as the Minions cavorted across his TV screen, he felt the comforting sameness of his daughter's love and he knew life would go on. Her laughter and a deep sense of gratitude began to heal the horror torn open by that morning's events.

His broken sense of self would become bigger, more expansive but it would take time. As the Minions played on, my exhausted truck driver floated into a deep and restful sleep and my work as a spirit, in the communion of all spirits, had begun.

Note from Nancy:

Gavin was my physical therapist a few years back. Helped me out when I had a bout of bursitis. I'd tell him about my conversations with the dead. He'd tell me about positive and negative energy, Karma and crystals. We agreed, we were both the 'nuttiest fruitcakes' the other had ever met. I think we both took it as a compliment.

Gavin's soul was the closest to an Atheist of any I ever encountered. I didn't understand all that DNA and 'epigenetic' intel his Angel imparted, but I suppose it makes as much sense as the cherubs, dead relatives, God and bright lights other folks encountered.

Toward the end of our conversations, even he was talking about the "communion of saints". I can't see cotton candy now without thinking of him and all those electron-infused nucleotides whizzing around among the living.

Leon's Story

*Suicide is man's way of telling God, 'You can't
fire me - I quit!'*

— Bill Maher

*Some people are just not meant to be in this
world. It's just too much for them.*

— Phoebe Stone

I heard the shot. I felt the heat of the bullet. Its momentum snapped my head back. I heard the crack of my skull as the bullet exited the back of my head. I heard the gun as it clattered across the floor. Then silence, a dark silence. I felt no pain, only the sensation of steely cold. And then, I was dead. The months before my suicide were an ever-steepening spiral of depression. I had received the eviction notice, telling me to get out of my little rental house. Three months before, I was fired from my job shitty job at the White Stone Senior Living Center. The month before that, I lost my only friend to a cancer. I was overweight, hypertensive, alone, drinking too much and usually stoned. It was as if the Universe was putting up neon signs that said, *"this way to the exit, no waiting!"* So, I just followed the signs. Pop! Dead.

Next thing I knew, I was reclining on a beach chair, overlooking a calm, light blue ocean with gently crashing waves and the hint of a refreshing breeze. I was wearing white board shorts that looked beautifully brilliant next to my tanned skin.

It was my skin that instantly grabbed my attention and for the first time in my life, I *wanted* to look in a mirror! My skin looked great. No blemishes anywhere. Not a single dimple of cellulite, no rolls of fat, not a hint of ashiness, just taunt muscle, glistening with a slight dewiness of perspiration.

What was even more delicious was the total absence of pain, anxiety and depression! I couldn't recall the last time I wasn't either hurting, frightened or sad. As I sat up, two tears, one from each eye, silently rolled down my cheeks and I felt them drip off my chin, onto my chest. Anxiety and depression, twin tears, literally rolled away.

In the distance, I could see a person, wearing khaki shorts, a blue baseball cap and a sparkling white tee shirt. He or she was walking towards me. Occasionally, this beach person would kick the surf, sending a spray of water into the air. Watching the droplets splash and return to the sand, my mind flashed back to my suicide.

As if in slow-motion, drops of falling ocean water morphed into blood, bits of bone and brains. I seemed to be watching from *inside* my body. I saw the contents of my skull splash against the wall. They splattered onto the curtains and across a cheap framed print showing the anatomy of the heart.

From my immobile body on the floor, I saw the nurse's feet as she opened the door of the examining room, and I heard her scream. Two more sets of feet, orderlies I guess, came running. The three of them tried to revive me, but I had researched my suicide and knew exactly where to shoot, what gun to use and the right ammo for maximum killing power. I was dead before I hit the floor, yet somehow, I was remembering everything in acute detail.

"Well, you can say what you want about your life, but your suicide was impeccable! Quite successful. Congratulations and welcome!"

The speaker, a handsome young guy, removed his cap with his left hand, bowed, extended his right hand to me. I instinctively shook it. He was lean and tanned. His longish brown hair was bushy from the ocean breeze and humidity. His white tee and khakis were impeccably neat, and he was smiling. He was in fact the kind of guy I fantasized about in my youth yet wouldn't have given me a second look.

"Was that a compliment?" I asked with a sly smile. (My god, I was flirting!)

"Kind of," he winked and sat on the foot of my beach chair. "I'm not condoning what you did but you did it well. Nice clean shot, right where the brain stem meets the foramen magnum!" He cocked his head back, closed his eyes, and with his right hand, index finger pointed as if holding a gun to the crease between his chin and neck, he made a sound like a ricocheting bullet, pa-ting!

"Some people botch the whole thing and linger for months on life support. Boring as hell! But" he slapped his thighs and sat up straight, "this isn't about other people! This is your chance to dish all the details: Why you did it, why you did it the *way* you did it, what pushed you over the edge? May I buy you a drink?"

I couldn't believe it! Barely stone-cold-dead and I was getting hit on in the afterlife! And he was cute, no less!

"Sure," I said with a smile. "What 'cha pouring?" It was a phrase my dad used to say, and it rolled off my tongue as if I'd been saying it forever. I hadn't.

"Everybody seems to like margaritas. Let's have one of those." He looked out over the ocean, and I followed his gaze. What appeared at first to be a bird, as big as a pelican, was slowly making its way toward us. As it neared, I heard a low hum and realized it was a drone, deftly delivering two large, frosty drinks garnished with lime wedges and salty rims.

My new Mr. McDreamy took one and gave the other to me. He raised his glass in my direction and said, "Here's to the best goddamn suicide we've ever seen!" We clinked glasses and savored our drinks.

I sat back and took a long pull off my margarita. "Ok," I said, "I did it because I couldn't envision a future I could endure, let alone be happy in. Everywhere I looked in my life, I was failing. Career, health, relationships, financially. I always seemed to be finishing last.

"The humiliation just became too much," I mumbled as I scanned the horizon. "That's it. No twisted stories about child abuse or deprivation. I was just defective when it came to coping. After 37 years of bad bets, I cashed out."

I drained off about half of what was left in my glass. Like magic, it refilled!

"Now, that's nifty!" I said as I raised my glass to admire its freshly replenished contents. "Free drinks in heaven, is it?" I asked.

"Ah, not exactly," my cute drinking buddy said. "The booze is free, but I don't think this is heaven, although it is nice. So, about the suicide? Why did you kill yourself in a hospital?"

"Oh, that! You know, I'm proud of this one! Nobody can say I didn't get this right," I said.

"I didn't want to do it in my house. The place was already a dump and me offing myself there would have made it even harder to clean up and rent. Violent death in a home is something realtors are required to disclose, and my old landlady had been nice to me."

"But why did you give a shit about her? I mean, you'd be dead!" Mr. McDreamy said.

I had to think for a minute, then I remembered. "I guess I just couldn't bear the thought of her finding my body," I said with a shrug.

"Ok, but a hospital? Why a hospital?" McDreamy asked.

"Well, since my house was out of the question, I needed a place. I thought about a public venue, like a library or a restaurant or a park, but that would really ruin those places for everyone who'd witness my suicide or stumbled across my body.

"I thought about a hotel room, but that didn't seem fair to the cleaning staff. I figured at a hospital, they'd be used to seeing death, and cleaning up blood and gore. I almost didn't do it there for fear they'd resuscitate me! So, I had to be sure to kill myself quickly and cleanly."

McDreamy's dark brown eyes were intently staring into mine. He nodded slightly as if encouraging me to continue.

"I bought the gun a week ago. I even took the course on how to hold it and fire the damn thing: A Colt King Cobra .357 Magnum, 6 Round Revolver. Small enough to grip firmly but powerful enough at close range to get the job done with the confidence I couldn't botch it.

"It was pricy, too! Nearly $900 for the gun and ammo. At first, I balked a little at having to buy a whole box of bullets. I mean, I only needed one, right? But then I realized I was putting everything on a credit card bill I would never have to pay, so what the fuck?" I raised my glass and polished off the rest of my margarita. Again, it refilled.

"When the clerk told me I should also buy shooting glasses and ear protection, I lied and told him I already had them. I mean, I couldn't tell him that my eye and ear health hardly mattered since I was going to kill myself!"

At this point, McDreamy piped up and said, "You should have gotten them! It'd be morbidly hilarious to find your head, blown to smithereens, sporting ear plugs and shooting glasses! Safety first, right?" He gave a double thumbs up and the cutest smile.

He continued, "So, how did you get your doctor to put you in the hospital?"

"The short answer is the opportunity simply presented itself. My cholesterol was dangerously high, so she scheduled a cardiac calcium scan and found I had a shit load of plaque in my arteries. Then, she scheduled an angiogram. It's a procedure where they inject your coronary arteries with dye and do an x-ray to look for blockages.

"The morning of my procedure, I put the gun in my backpack and just walked into the hospital's heart clinic. I got undressed, put on the little open-in-the-back cotton gown, sat on the exam table and blew my brains out."

Mr. McDreamy mumbled something about how I should have waited for the angiogram results, "I mean, if you'd only waited a month or two, you could've saved the price of the gun and ammo and let your heart kill you," he chuckled.

We sat in silence again until McDreamy said, "We'll, thanks for the explanation." He then stretched and yawned, patted my leg and whispered, "I need to think. Enjoy your margarita," and with that he sat cross-legged on the sand next to me, sipping his drink while staring out over the sea.

What the fuck? If I'd known suicide was a ticket to a booze-laden-beach Paradise, with a hunky guy, I'd have blown my brains out years ago! Everything around me was perfect! The temperature, the light, the setting, my budding relationship with Mr. McDreamy! I had this rocking body and I felt great!

Maybe it was the bottomless margarita. Maybe it was the release from the stress I'd been carrying for so long in life, but everything around me, the ocean waves, the breeze, began to slow down and swirl. I drifted into a deep, comfy slumber and began to dream.

In my dream, I could hear indistinct voices, lots of them. They were talking, laughing, sometimes shouting. It was the background noise of a massive arena or theatre, just before the show. As my eyes adjusted to the darkened space, I saw that it was, in fact a college lecture hall with a lectern, set up in a spotlight on the well below. Every now and then, I picked up snippets of words and sentences:

"Who cares? We're dead, right? Hahahaha!"

"Suicide by the sewer's side? Hysterical!

"Da, da, da, da, da, da, da, dead man!" to the tune of the Batman theme.

All the hubbub continued until my Mr. McDreamy walked out into the pool of light at the lectern. He was wearing a tux. He stood behind the lectern and said into the slightly crackling microphone, "Ok, take your seats. Settle down. Act unlively," and at this, a corporate chuckle undulated across the assembled throng. With growing attention, we all settled down and turned toward the lectern.

"Congratulations on successfully quitting life and welcome to your next…ah, ad… adventure. You are officially dead." And with that there were some scattered applause and some equally scattered gasps and groans."

"I know, "continued McDreamy in a mock-weary voice, "some of you were just *trying* to *almost* commit suicide. Well, consider yourself to have finally overachieved!" Again, a smattering of weak laughter.

"I'll be brief. The first order of business is to sort yourselves…Christians, over here, Muslims, over here. Buddhist, here…." This went on for a while as all the souls shuffled into place by religious or spiritual beliefs.

Now, I had been raised a Christian but when that tribe shunned me for being queer, I gave up on church. I was probably 15, maybe a little older. I'd read a lot about different religions but didn't seem to fit any of them, so I just went and stood with the "other" crowd.

McDreamy pulled a small notebook from his inside breast pocket and began reading:

72

"Christians. Listen up! You tell each other that God abhors suicide because it destroys His most perfect creation. Yet, nowhere in the Bible is suicide explicitly called out as a sin, as opposed to adultery, theft, and idolatry. You know the spiel."

There was some mumbling and nodding among the Christians.

"It does, however, fall into some categories of sinful behavior, like committing murder or the hubris of thinking one knows better than God. In short, your Bible is a big ole sack of contradictions! Y'all need to spend some time with God to hash this out." And with that, all the Christians vanished.

"Jews? Where are my Jews? Always wandering!" Again, some scattered laughter. McDreamy was remarkably good at this emcee gig!

"Ok, if killing others is sinful, surely whacking oneself is! That's what Orthodox Jews say. "However," and here, McDreamy raised a finger and paused for effect, "the Jewish legal standard for suicide stipulates that those who take their own lives because of mental illness, are exempt from any repercussions in the hereafter. And let's face it," McDreamy said with a knowing grin, "All of you were pretty mentally fucked up when you were offing yourselves, so get out of here, you crazy Jews, and go enjoy eternity!" At last, I thought to myself, the Jews finally caught a break!

"Now, the Buddhist? Okay! Your beliefs on suicide are almost neutral. I mean, you guys know you're going to die and be reincarnated anyway, so what's the point? There is, however, the pesky bit about killing, which you are not supposed to do. You cannot have it both ways, Buddhist! Go noodle this out among yourselves.

Muslims! Suicide is bad, full stop.... unless you're martyring yourself, in which case, it's Allah's good graces, a Crown of Dignity and eternal life all around! My advice?" And with that, McDreamy lowering his voice, he cocked his right eyebrow, and put his mouth right next to the microphone. In a whispery, conspiratorial voice, he said, "Just say you did it for the glory of Allah and you should be fine."

Well, this went on for a good long while until a few Wicca practitioners, an Atheist and I were the only ones left. And Wicca? Well, according to McDreamy, Wiccans die (it doesn't matter how) when their purpose on earth is finished. They believe they go to the Wiccan Summerland, a place of plenty and contentment, where they await their next incarnation.

Frankly, my experience on the beach seemed a lot like the Summerland: Warm sun, a comfortable chair, sparkling blue ocean, white sand, a cute dude and unlimited margaritas.

Somewhere in the distance, I heard a noise I couldn't quite make out. Bagpipes?

I awoke, still in my beach chair as my khaki-shorts companion seemed to be working out a rendition of "Come on Baby Light my Fire," that looked and sounded like a cat fight! He was indeed playing the bagpipes!

"Ah, could you stop that?" I raised my voice a little and said it again.

"I could, but I won't," McDreamy replied out the corner of his mouth. He piped on. After a while, he said, "I told you this isn't Heaven. It's a *kind* of paradise, alright, but it has its limits.

For instance," and he held up the flopping pipes, "when I asked for a musical instrument, I wanted a guitar. These bagpipes showed up. When I asked for a beer, I got a margarita. Same with my request for Chardonnay, a screwdriver or a martini: Margarita, every time."

McDreamy fingered the bagpipes and continued. "We're stuck on this beautiful beach. We have no money, no clothes other than what we are wearing and it's just us, nobody else. We have nothing to eat, but we'll never get hungry. Go figure."

He went back to his bagpipes. This time the song was, I think, Purple Rain. When he finished the tune, (the only way I could tell he'd finish was because he simply quit playing) I asked, "Please, tell me more about where we are and what I should expect. And," (was I blushing?) "I'd like to know a little about you."

The bagpipes groaned pathetically as he laid them on the sand, where they slowly disintegrated. With a reverence and solemnity, I'd never experienced in life, Mr. McDreamy, took both my hands. He pulled me up to stand in front of him.

Looking into my eyes, he said, "Honey, I am you."

For a long time, we just stared at each other. I slowly began to recognize myself, my perfect self, standing before me. It was like looking in a mirror, but refreshingly, without any self-loathing. Where I used to see a smallish head, narrow shoulders, wide hips and cellulite, I now saw a rather ordinary man who was at peace with himself, standing tall, smiling and beautiful.

The person I had first seen as a handsome hunk, the person I'd wanted to "hit on me," to love me...was me.

"You may think you've just committed suicide, but the truth is, you killed me, this part of you, a long time ago. I was the little boy who wanted to dance, to pretend he was Jeannie and Samantha from TV. You were ashamed of me, embarrassed by me! I could have helped you and saved us from suicide if you'd only loved me."

"Instead, you just denied me and tried to please everyone else. And I'm pretty pissed about it, too!" McDreamy-me was now staring me down, close to tears but defiant.

"I'm sorry," I said, but something about the man before me gave me the courage to add, "You did embarrass me. You got me beaten up more times than I can remember. I didn't know how to love you! That whole Golden Rule thing about loving others as you love yourself? I never understood it! I felt like I could love others, but I couldn't find anything about myself, about you, to love!"

"So now, in death, it's come down to just us," McDreamy said, "just us, you and me. Trying to sort out our shattered soul and become one with, what? God? The Universe? Who knows? So far, it's just been me waiting for you, walking on an endless beach, playing the bagpipes and drinking margaritas."

For what seemed like ages, we just stared into each other's faces and talked. "Why do you suppose you never loved yourself?" McDreamy said. He was smiling slightly, still holding my hands.

It was a question many therapists had posed to me. I had been criticized, ridiculed and neglected a lot in my infancy and youth. It wasn't that my parents hated me, although they took every opportunity to tell me and everyone within earshot that I was unplanned, a mistake, a surprise. They just didn't have the energy or money to raise another kid.

"If you really are me, you already know the answer," I said. "Financially, emotionally, I was a bother. I grew up assuming I was bad, stupid and a nuisance. Pour atop that the fact that I grew up a gay boy in a small town. My sister was a beauty queen, my brother was a straight A student, and I was just…there, an embarrassing little faggot, taking up space and scarce resources: Always in the way, always needing something at the most inopportune time. It got a little better as I grew up, moved away and started my own life but I couldn't shake the feeling that I was an imposter, pretending to be somebody, when everyone around me was laughing at me behind my back!"

"Oh, your paranoia was justified," McDreamy said with a snide laugh, "but only because you spent an awful lot of energy trying to be something you were not. Honey, we were gayer than a pussy-pink purse at a Pride Parade! You just never understood that loving me, us, was the ticket out."

"I didn't know how to love you!" I screamed in hot anger. "I mean, at times you were totally unlovable!"

"Go on," McDreamy said with a sneer.

"Okay…" I said slowly. The feelings of shame and humiliation were welling up in me like a growing tidal wave. "Like that time *you* agreed that we would be the 'bride' in the womanless wedding skit for Boy Scouts. It wasn't enough for you to drape a towel around your waist and use a dish rag as a veil! No! You had to take our mother's wedding dress from the attic, slap on a dime store wig and finish it off with lipstick!"

"Somehow, we convinced ourself that this was a theatrical role. You said all the girl parts were played by men in Shakespeare's time. You actually had me believing we could pull this off!

"So, I show up at the Presbyterian Church fellowship hall, in bugger drag! At first, the other boys tell me I have a hilarious costume. 'I'm thinking, this is great!' Then, I start to pick up on the snide remarks and the mocking whispers. My parents sat in the audience, mortified and when it was all over the other scouts beat me up in the cloakroom and took turns pretending to bugger me in the ass! That was 4th grade and it stuck with me all the way through high school!"

McDreamy hung his head in what I took to be remorse. When he at last looked at me, though, his face was contorted in rage.

"You poor, dumb, bastard," he said enunciating each word. "If you'd only *owned it*, we could have pulled it off!

79

If only you'd swished in and said, 'Yeah, I'm way prettier than any girl who will ever give any of you assholes the time of day!' And yes, I admit, I should have taken off the wedding dress and the lipstick before going to the punch and cookies reception in the fellowship hall, but the fact is, even though I knew I was going to get beaten up, in that moment, *I felt pretty and I liked the way I looked!*"

Another long, awkward silence.

Finally, I said to McDreamy, "You mean, if I'd just accepted…."

"No! Not accepted! Embraced!" McDreamy's eyes were tearing up and his voice got louder. "We're smart and handsome. We are articulate and witty and way too compassionate for our own good. In fact, you let the frightened, cringing part of us take over, making me, the beautiful, flamboyant, charming queer, smaller and smaller."

McDreamy was getting angry. He started pacing. "You always took less and put others first. You practically groveled to the straight folks, craving their approval. You minimized *me* into non-existence! You didn't even assert our dignity in death! Killing yourself in a hospital, to make it easy on the people who would have to clean up the mess? That's pathetic"

"I was only trying to be considerate," I mumbled.

"Be honest," McDreamy-me said. "You were trying to be *invisible*, even in death. Hell, I'm surprised you didn't just find a dumpster behind the hospital, close the lid and *then* blow our brains out! They could have just dumped the body in the landfill! Or, what the heck? Even better, you could've just blown our head off, in the middle of the goddamn landfill, at midnight!

You always hid me, telling me it was safer to hide, whisper and walk softly. I wanted to come out! Sing out loud in public, strut! But your fear of rejection and ridicule held me back. *You killed me long ago!*"

McDreamy just stared into my eyes with smoldering anger. He was so beautiful and strong. Not tough-guy strong, more like the kind of moral strength that comes from being right.

And then, I did something I'd never done before. I confronted my big old gay self and said, "you're absolutely right." Before I even thought about it, I took him into my arms, "I'm so sorry," I whispered, "you embarrassed me, and I was afraid of you."

I instantly felt bigger. I felt more like a protector than ever before. I was overcome with love and appreciation for the man I was, not the man I wished I was or the pitiful, ugly person I thought myself to be.

"I love you," I said.

"And I love you," said McDreamy. "But love isn't enough." Our embrace ended. McDreamy took my hand and led me along the beach, our feet lightly splashing in the surf.

"I don't understand," I said. "If love isn't enough, what is?"

McDreamy didn't answer. He just smiled and cast his gaze down the beach.

"So where is everyone?" I asked. Apart from a beach chair, flying margaritas, one set of disappearing bagpipes, and my dream featuring the planet's religions, I'd seen no evidence of anything or anyone else. "Where's God?"

"I'm as clueless as you are," said McDreamy-me, "but I have a theory: When I found you on the beach, I knew you were me, but you didn't recognize that I was you. That's because you had suppressed me to the point that I was unrecognizable! I think we are here to put ourself back together, no matter how long it may take and only you…we can do it."

"Is this the punishment for suicide, maybe?" I asked?

"I don't think so," said McDreamy. "We're just here, together, for some kind of cosmic time-out, maybe to reflect on life and give it another go?"

"Well, aren't you the deep thinker?" I said with a smile.

"And you are, too," laughed McDreamy. "If I think it, *you* think it, too. We just need to get all of us in sync. No more repression!"

"Maybe suicide is just life's way of miscarrying?" I mused. "I mean, for whatever reasons, we didn't develop properly. We failed to thrive. We just weren't...viable. To be honest, I figured we were bound for horns and pitchforks!"

"No, I think the Universe is more forgiving than that," said McDreamy. "What kind of Supreme Being would put a tortured soul into more agony? I think we must assume we are here for a purpose and that purpose begins with us becoming equals, who respect ourself. We must do that before we get around to love."

I added randomly, "Do you suppose there is a God?"

"I do," McDreamy responded. "I mean, something has to be responsible for all this," he said as he motioned between us and then all around to our unlimited beach."

"Or" I mused, "Maybe this is just what happens to everybody who commits suicide? Maybe this is loser heaven," I chuckled.

When McDreamy didn't respond, I looked into his face and saw the red-hot cheeks of humiliation. "You're still doing it." He whispered. *We. Are. Not. A. Loser!"*

The words were fierce, spoken as a growl, through gritted teeth. "Stop trying to pass every slight, every insult off as a joke! It's not a joke! We're dead because you would not stand up for us and admit *we are gay, and we are angry*! You killed us because you were afraid to demand dignity! You killed us in the hope that, just maybe in death, you could end the self-hatred. Well, guess what? I still hate you!"

He yelled so forcefully, so loudly, I could almost see vibrations coming out of his mouth!

As quickly as my brawny-strong-protector feelings had come, they rapidly fizzled. Once again, I was a split second away from groveling and apologizing for having an opinion when McDreamy smiled and said…

"Oh, *God*, that felt good!" And suddenly, I felt it, too. He…I, had literally stood up to myself, stood up for myself, and there was no one here to make me regret it! This wasn't "loser heaven" but it wasn't exactly any other kind of heaven, either.

As if finishing my thought, McDreamy said, "Whatever it is, we're the only ones here. Besides, lots of people who were far from being losers committed suicide. Cleopatra, Nero, Meriweather Lewis, Sylvia Plath, Robin Williams…I don't see any of them here."

"Do you think all the suicides get our own private beach," I mused. "Just imagine, if we had multiple personality disorder, we could have our own baseball team!"

84

"Very funny," McDreamy chuckled, "as if any of our multiple personalities would even want to play baseball. But, what now?"

McDreamy continued to answer his rhetorical question. "I'm pretty sure there is a God around here somewhere, but for now, looks like it's just you and me," and then he added, "I think we just have to put ourselves back together again, Humpty-Dumpty."

And with that, my confident, McDreamy-self draped an arm across my shoulders, looked out over the light blue sea and said, "This is going to take a while. Want a margarita?"

Note from Nancy:

Leon and I talked many times over the years, both before and after his death. He took getting fired from the nursing home hard, even though it wasn't his fault. It was just numbers. Whenever a few of us died off, they simply didn't need as many attendants!

Being Leon, he took it personally. Said he thought it was because he was gay. Turns out, Leon attributed every bad thing that had ever happened to him as a direct result of being a homo! That's when I came out to Leon!

And let me just say to all the straight folk out there, National Coming Out Day is fine and dandy, but in reality, the queer folk in your life come out all the time! Every time we get to know someone or make a new friend, the conversation goes something like this:

Straight Woman: "Are you married?"

Me: "Widowed."

SW: "Oh, me too. How long has your husband been gone?"

Me: "I had a wife. She's been gone 17 years."

At this point the new acquaintance looks surprised, and I'm left wondering if that is an 'oh shit' surprised look or a 'that's cool' look of surprise. If it's the former, the conversion usually comes to a rapid close with the straight person making a mumbled excuse about something urgently requiring his or her attention. If it's the latter, the getting-to-know-you process moves on and you find other things you have in common or interests you both might share: ex.:

"I always wanted to go skydiving."

"Really? Me to! What are you doing next Thursday?"

In other words, one's sexuality or gender identity shouldn't define one's existence. It's just one in a myriad of traits that make us who we are.

Leon saw his gayness as a flaw. It was a defect he spent his whole life trying to alternately fix or hide. It was during one of our Hooligan conversations that I explained how I had come to terms with being a big old southern lesbian. It seemed to help. I share it now, in the hopes that some poor gay soul will read it and skip the whole rigmarole Leon had to go through in reclaiming his soul in Heaven.

I had known from the beginning that I was way more boyish than girlie, more of a tree climber and less of a baby-doll hugger. It wasn't that I wanted to be a boy. I just liked boy things growing up and the older I got, I was especially attracted to girls is a crushy, romantic sort of way.

I understood Leon's angst and like almost every queer kid in the world, I had felt it, too: That sneaky suspicion something was "different" about me. That's where my experience and Leon's diverged. I didn't think my identity was wrong or bad. I just knew I was different. As I reached puberty, I didn't quite fit the mold society and my straight girlfriends were settling into. I didn't know any girls like me. Hell, I was grown before I even knew there was a name for it!

The fact is, I didn't come out to myself until I was almost 40 and divorced. It finally dawned on me that I was being dishonest! By failing to honor my true self, my honest desire to love a woman, I wasn't living up to my full potential. I was like a dog walking around on its hind legs. It was possible, it was ok, but it wasn't...the real me!

I think my friend Betty said it best. When I asked Betty about her life with a husband and two wives (all in three different, monogamous relationships, thank God) she told me to think of it this way: She said, "Champagne is good, but did you ever notice that it just tastes better when you drink it out of a long-stemmed crystal flute? The very same champagne will not taste as good in an old tin cup." And that," she continued, "is the way I always looked at sexuality! With a man, it was ok, even better if you were in love. But sex with a woman? Oh, for me, that was champagne in a crystal goblet!" God, I miss Betty.

I think Leon was coming out to himself on that beach. He'd spent almost his whole life on earth obsessed with trying to not be gay only to discover that, even in death, we cannot escape who we really are.

Frankie's Story

When you change the way you look at things, the things you look at change.

-Dr. Wayne Dyer

We must be willing to let go of the life we planned so as to have the life that is waiting for us.

-Joseph Campbell

"Surprise!"

The word rang out and echoed as party noisemakers bleated amid more cheers of "surprise." Balloons and confetti fell all around me as a spotlight from somewhere high above snapped on with a ka-thunk, a low hum and the brightest glow I'd ever seen.

As the noise faded and the light softened, I began to make out the forms of faces, all smiling and looking right at me. For as far as I could see, there was an ocean of what looked like black and white, life-sized cut outs…of people! I was standing right in the middle of them, bathed in a pool of white light.

The first one I recognized was my maternal grandmother. In life, all her grandchildren called her Mama. She had twinkling eyes and the most generous, beatific smile. Her plump face framed by beautiful gray curls, expertly coiffed once a week by Miss Mary at the beauty shop. She was exactly as I remembered, wearing a simple house dress and an apron. Without even thinking, I reached out and lightly touched her image.

"Oh, there's my girl!" Speaking these words, she blossomed into full color and became real! I stumbled back a few steps and bumped into another of the cut outs behind me and my dead-husband, Bob, sprang to life, wearing his trademark fishing hat, dappled with flies he'd tied himself.

"Hey, settle down, girl," he said with a crooked smile. "It's just us!"

"Who?" I managed to sputter.

Mama wrapped her arms around me and said, "Everyone you've ever loved and lost. Surprise!"

I started scanning the black and white faces surrounding us. There was my maternal grandfather, my paternal grandparents, my parents. Pets. Pets! Every hamster, horse, dog and cat I'd ever known was there, just as I remembered them. I realized I was smiling and the only word I could muster was, "What?"

Mama and Dead Bob smiled and looked up into the light. "Well, that, up there is where we came from. And this," Bob indicated the immobile crowd around us, "is your welcoming committee! So far, it's just me and Mama here but you'll eventually get around to everybody."

Bob took me in his arms and for a moment, we hugged, then kissed. He looked deeply into my eyes and with the kindest, most loving voice, he said, "it's so good to be held like you're really loved, isn't it?" Missing his kiss, his touch, was the greatest longing I had ever known. The only thing I can liken it to is the ache of homesickness.

Bob had died five years before, when his flu turned into pneumonia. It was as if a chunk of me had been torn out and left to heal with no treatment, no way to kill the pain. Holding him, seeing him again was like a soothing balm, flooding into the raw emptiness.

"But this is a surprise," Bob continued.

And Mama chimed in, "We weren't expecting you quite so soon."

Mama kissed my cheek and squeezed my hand. "Just look at you! You look just like your mother," she said, pointing at another cutout that did, indeed looked a lot like me. It was my mother, exactly as she was the last time I saw her, only smiling and looking...joyful? Yes, the look on her face was beyond mere happiness. It was a gracious, mischievous bliss, as if she had a secret she couldn't wait to tell!

"This is a dream," I mumbled to myself.

"You will probably call it that when you tell the story," Mama said, "but it's more of an altered reality. You see, that light up there is a gateway, a passage into our next existence."

"Heaven? God?" I whispered as if I didn't want to be overheard."

"Call it whatever you want," Bob chuckled. "Here, in this reality, you can enliven anyone or anything from your life to this point, provided they're dead. Everyone here is exactly as *you* remember them. See, this right here, is just a way station, a waiting room for the not-quite-dead, like you.

But, once you're dead-dead," Bob continued, "you get to move fluidly into any time in your previous life. I usually stay somewhere around eight or nine years old and, as you might guess," he pointed to his hat, "I spend most of my time fishing."

92

"Go ahead. Ask Granddaddy," Mama said, and she pointed to her husband, grinning and immobile by her side.

I touched his hand and instantly he grabbed mine and pulled me in for a hug. "Come here, you little monkey!" He growled. "Course, you're not so little anymore. How old are you," He asked.

I had to think for a moment. "Fi-Fifty-seven," I stammered.

"Well, you're still cute as a dad-gum button," he chuckled as he patted my head and continued, "We sure didn't expect to see you here for a good long time, did we Mama?"

"Oh, I think not," Mama cooed.

"So where is here and what is happening?" I said, still totally unable to process the experience.

Bob was the first to speak up, "Like Mama said, the next life awaits you, but you are here way early. Seems you've been allowed a little visit. You've been granted the opportunity to 'touch' a few of us who, in life, touched you."

"I, don't understand, "I said, near panic. "Help me," I cried.

Instantly, Bob, Mama, Grandaddy and I were sitting in the rocking chairs on the side porch of Mama's and Granddaddy's old home place. It had been gone for decades but here we were, on what seemed to be a summer afternoon. Across the road, I could see the peach shed. The smell of fresh peaches from my granddaddy's north Georgia orchards filled the air. There were red and yellow roses on the trellises and iris blooming, somehow totally out of season, in the garden with azaleas and hydrangeas also in full bloom. Mama had a lap full of string beans from a bushel basket next to her chair. She was snapping the beans and throwing them into a big, glazed bowl.

"Honey, you've had a concussion," she said as she snapped away. Using her foot, she pushed the bushel of beans toward me and indicated I should start snapping, too.

"Do you remember what you were up to just before you saw us?" She asked.

At first, I did not. Then, Bob prompted, "You'd left your office to get lunch at the Chinese Bistro on Lexington Ave. near East 54th Street."

The name of the place, Lexington Avenue, triggered a flash of recollection. I could faintly smell basil and garlic. Takeout in hand, I grabbed a fortune cookie from the jar by the door. The bell on the door jingled and I exited the bistro.

As I stepped out onto the sidewalk, something big came barreling into my field of peripheral vision and slammed into me with such force! The last thing I could recall was a painful bump from the left, watching my takeout food flying off to the right, and my head hitting the pavement with a crack.

"Yeah…" I said with a soft exhale. "What was that all about?"

"We'll, from what I could surmise from the chatter of the EMTs," Bob said excitedly, "you stepped out in front of a rather large man on an electric bike, riding down the sidewalk. He's going to be ok. If you live, he'll be charged with a misdemeanor but if you die, he will likely face involuntary manslaughter charges."

"So, you see," Grandaddy said as pulled a Kent cigarette from the pack in his shirt pocket, "if you don't go back, you're going to miss out on the rest of your life and most likely mess up his life too."

I looked at Grandaddy and then back at Bob and whispered, "There's smoking in Heaven?"

"Not really, Bob said. "You've had a concussion. Your memories and imagination are scrambled. You remember him as a smoker, so that's how he is. Stay focused on what's happening, not the details. He's saying, if you stay here before your time, there will be consequences."

"But I have a choice?" I asked no one in particular. Bob spoke first. "It, it's, a…hard to say," he stuttered a little, implying uncertainty and sadness.

"In my case, my lungs were so far gone that my body couldn't have taken me back. I tried! I really didn't want to leave you, but it was my time."

"Same with Mama and me, "Granddaddy said. "I don't know how long I was here without her..."

"Nearly 3 years," I said.

"Well, whatever it was, when we saw each other again, it was as if nothing had changed," Mama said and the look between them was full of the kind of intimacy that comes from decades of love and mutual admiration.

"The thing is," Mama continued, looking back at her lap-full of beans, "every now and then, something happens, and someone shows up here long before their time," and then she looked at Grandaddy and mused, "maybe it's sorta like when your plane gets in early and there's no available gate or the jetway is missing?"

"Or maybe it's sort of a cosmic catch and release," Bob offered.

"Or" Granddaddy chimed in, "we're just a delusion God has planted in your head to help you figure out a few things while the rest of your brain is on autopilot."

"The fact is," Bob continued, "we just don't know. We don't know exactly where we are, but for the three of us, it's...home. We don't know if this is eternal or just a phase. We don't even know if there's a God calling the shots, but we are pretty darn sure some powerful force is running this show."

"What I do know," said Grandaddy as he lit his cigarette, "is that it is so good to see you!" And he patted my knee.

"And it's good to see all of you, too," I gushed, "and I want to go back to that place where I came in and see everyone! I want to talk to my parents, my other Grandparents. I want to see Shep and Bowzer, KitKat, Star and all the other dogs, cats and horses we had!" And I looked at Bob and blurted out, "This is the first time since you died that I haven't felt…empty."

Grandaddy, Mama and Bob exchanged glances, as if they knew something I didn't. And they surely did.

Grandaddy smoked his Kent for what seemed like the longest time. Mama and I snapped beans and Bob fiddled with the flies on his hat. We just talked about people, peaches, flowers in the garden. We were all laughing at one of Bob's fish stories when I popped open a bean and a small, rolled up piece of paper fell out. Everyone fell silent.

"Go on," Mama said, not looking up from her beans. "It's not going to read itself."

The paper was a little shorter than my thumb and sure enough, when I unrolled it, there was a message. It said: *Nothing has changed. Everything is different.*

"Nothing has changed. Everything is different." I read it again, this time, aloud. "What kind of bean-fortune is that supposed to be?" I whispered to no one in particular.

"Oh, that's no fortune cookie," Bob said excitedly. "It's the answer to why you've been feeling so empty since I died."

"You see," Bob explained, "I died, but life and the business of living went on. People went to work. Our friends kept doing the same stuff they'd always done, all as if nothing had changed, because for them, nothing really had changed. Yet for you, *everything was different*! My place at the table, my dirty clothes basket, my side of the bed. All empty, right? That was the visible emptiness. The emptiness is your heart is what you're still feeling."

"And, if I stay here, the emptiness goes away?" It was more of a wish than a question.

"There's only one way to get rid of emptiness," Mama said, quietly as she patted my arm. "You just gotta go back and fill it up!"

Somewhere, beyond the peach shed and past the orchards, I became aware of a faint, persistent beeping noise, like a garbage truck, backing up.

"Mama's right," said Grandaddy. He stood up and walked to the edge of the porch and deftly rolled his cigarette butt between his fingers until the ember at the tip fell to the gravel beside the porch. Then he put the remaining filter in his pocket. He called it "field stripping", a technique he learned in the Army during WWII. Perhaps this little visit was my subconscious, field stripping the grief from my soul?

"Go back, "Bob whispered. "Heck, we'll still be here when you finally die. We aren't going anywhere! Remember, *nothing has changed*. All those folks, your animals you saw earlier, we'll all be right here. You just go back now and make a new life, fill it, make it different."

The beeping noise was growing louder and there was a ringing behind it now. Slowly, the porch scene was fading. Mama and Grandaddy were gone and, where my Bob had been, there stood a precious little brown-haired boy, wearing an impossibly big fishing hat.

"Nothing has changed. Everything is different," he said with a grin and a shrug. "I'm still me and one day, we'll be together again. But right now, you have empty spaces to fill with life and love. You need to heal that concussion. Nothing has changed. Go live. Love. Be the light in someone else's life. I'll be right here when you get back."

Gently, my little-boy-Bob squeezed my hand and ran off, behind the peach shed, through the orchard and presumably to the farm pond in the valley below.

And with that, I felt the most excruciating pain I had ever known. I couldn't move my head! I couldn't move at all! Somehow, I realize that my inability to move was because my body was strapped down and my head was wedged between some kind of blocks. I was in an ambulance, siren blaring.

The beeping I had heard earlier was a heart monitor. Someone pulled open my right eyelid and I faintly heard the words, "pupils" and "responsive". Whoever said it seemed happy with that.

I was about to go back, into my life, and except for a concussion and a fractured hip, nothing had changed, yet from that day forward, everything was different.

Note from Nancy:

This was the only time I ever spoke to someone who didn't stay dead!

I'd met Frankie and her grandmother at the nursing home years ago. I guess Mama told Frankie about the Hooligan because somehow, in death (or near death) Frankie found me and told me her story just before she came back. I knew where she worked and sent her some little get-well flowers during her recovery. She acknowledged the gift but apparently had no recollection of our little tete-a-tete via the Hooligan. Last I heard, she'd left her corporate job in

New York, moved back to her hometown in North Georgia and remarried.

The weirdest thing? In her thank you note acknowledging the flowers, Frankie told me one of the EMT's had found the fortune cookie she snatched on the way out of the Asian Bistro, clutched in her hand. She saved it for her and delivered it to her while she was still in the hospital. Apparently, Frankie crushed the cookie in her fist when she fell to the pavement.

Inside was a fortune, printed on a slip of paper, a little smaller than your thumb. It read, "You will live long and open many fortune cookies."

Adam's Story

Teach your parents well. Their children's hell will
slowly go by.

- Graham Nash

Forgiveness is the fragrance the violet sheds on the
heel that crushed it.

-Mark Twain

Technically, every father is a motherfucker, right? I mean, he wouldn't be your father unless he fucked your mother.

This little epiphany popped into my brain the instant after it was flooded with blood from a massive aneurysm. It was as if a fire hydrant exploded in the center of my head and the first thought that gushed out was one of pure hatred for my dad.

I'd just finished a set of mixed doubles at the country club. One minute, there I was chatting away, a cold, sweaty glass of iced tea in hand, and the next, my body crumpled to the ground, dead. And now, I'm standing…somewhere, still wearing my tennis togs, contemplating motherfuckery? Where'd that come from?

Then, as if that wasn't weird enough, the biggest MFer of them all was walking right towards me! My dad emerged through billowing clouds of white smoke, but there was no smell of anything burning. No smell of anything at all. No noise of footsteps. I heard my own voice saying, "Dad? Is that you?"

The question carried anxiety and even a little fear. I mean, if my gaping anus of a father was here, *here* most certainly was not heaven! Seeing the look on my face, Dad smiled that familiar sarcastic smirk and said, "Not the Heavenly Father you expected, huh?"

I was still staring at him as he walked right past me and sat in one of two nearby hefty, white wooden Adirondack chairs, just like the ones we used to have in the backyard when I was a kid.

This was the man who had abused me, mentally and physically. After my mother's death, I went into foster care.

I would go years at a time without laying eyes on him, only to have him show up unexpectedly, at my school, college, later my work, usually drunk (sometimes just hungover and shaky) and always needing money.

Often, he was homeless, disheveled, dirty. But the person before me now looked great! He was rested, fit, well-groomed, clean. He wore a white tee shirt, light gray suit and gray loafers. He looked…dapper?

I last saw him at my med school graduation. Amid the caps and gowns, the blooming dogwoods and azaleas, the mid-May finery of boutonnières and pastel linen sport coats, there he was, wearing a filthy yellow track suit and brown rubber flip flops.

He was totally wasted. His face was grubby, unshaven, and he was waving a lit cigarette (in a smoke-free arena, of course). His underarms were stained with stale sweat and peeking from his pants pocket was the top of a brown pint bottle of something, no doubt cheap and alcoholic.

When they called my name, he shouted, "Way to go, you little pussy! Hey! Now, you can be your own gynecologist!" A couple of security guards quietly escorted him from the arena. That was 5 years ago. About three years after that, I heard he died, in jail, broke. I didn't know where he was buried and didn't care.

My first instinct was to walk away. I tried, yet each time I walked into the clouds, I would remember some horrible thing he'd done and emerge again to see him in that chair, sitting silently and staring straight ahead. It was as if every memory led back to him.

There was the time I'd rushed into the living room on Christmas morning to find him passed out drunk, atop a half-assembled bike. The time he came out into the basketball court, in the middle of the game and slapped my seven-year-old face for missing a free throw. The time at age 9 when I spent the night in a Waffle House because he forgot to pick me up after baseball practice.

Once, he got arrested for driving drunk and without a license. I was in the car, eleven years old. I spent that night on the floor of the police station, waiting for him to sober up and be let out of jail.

He'd beat my mother, steal from her and me (I learned early not to leave loose change around). There were so many broken promises, missed birthdays, too many punches, jeers and verbal abuses to recall exactly but they were all seared into my soul. And they all led back to the embarrassment, anguish and disappointment that defined the memories of my father.

The funny thing was these memories didn't make me sad or even angry anymore. I was just numb. Maybe this is what it means to be dead: A lack of any emotion, a numbness we seek but can't find in life?

"Are you done yet?" It was his voice, but somehow there was an unfamiliarity to it. It was softer, less gravelly than I recalled. "You're dead wrong, ya know. Ha! Dead wrong. Get it?

"Uh?" I eloquently replied.

"Your conclusion about death and numbness."

"What?" Again, I understood the words but how did he know what I was thinking?

"Are you done ticking off all the times I hurt you? All the slights and brutishness? I know it's what you're doing. Not my first rodeo."

"What?" I said again.

"Look, I know you're trying to get your head around what's going on here but if all you can muster are single syllable inquiries, this is going to require a lot of guesswork on my part. So, let me go first: Do you have any idea what's going on here?"

I shook my head no.

"So, we've gone from one word communication to sign language? Jesus, son. Sit down." He pointed to the other chair and without question, I did as I was asked.

"What's the last thing you remember before seeing me?" Again, his voice was calm, silky even, and the look on his face was something I'd rarely seen before: his clear, focused, undivided attention.

"I was in the club house," I said. "Given the pain in my head, I'd say I blew an aneurysm." Then, realizing I was having a conversation with the king of MFers, I quickly shot back, "And why would you care?" I asked, not as much in anger but in genuine curiosity.

"Oh, I've always cared!" He patted my knee and chuckled. "I was just too broken and addicted to show it. You were too young and victimized to understand. By the time you were old enough to appreciate the situation, I was eaten up with cirrhosis and you'd built a wall of denial around yourself. Inside your reality, I was the villain who killed your mother and abandoned you. Now, I'm dead, you're dead and your little fantasy wall is about to come crashing down. Funny, how life caved in on us both…you with hate and me with addiction."

When I said nothing, he continued. It was as if I were watching a movie or a play: A one man-show for a one-man audience.

"Congratulations on beating the cycle of addiction and abuse, by the way. My dad, my granddaddy, they were all abusive, addicted boozers. Thanks to a little popped vein-bubble in your brain, you're the end of the line! By the way," he added casually, "you never took a single drink in your whole life. Not one sip, not one puff of weed, nothing."

"I couldn't stand the smell of beer, wine, weed or liquor, thanks to you! Seeing someone high disgusted me. I knew their escape from reality was ruining another life or lives somewhere. So, thanks for being such a jerk! You can take credit for childlessness and my sobriety."

"And you never dated much, never fell in love, got married?" He asked.

I just told him the truth. "I was afraid I'd be a terrible husband and dad. Like you."

He seemed unmoved by my confession. Calm even. All I could do was stare at his face: mesmerized by how great he looked and at the same time revolted by the memories.

"What's going on here," Dad explained, "is sort of what they do in AA. I'm apologizing. I'm sorry. Your hating me is understandable and I wish things had been different. I was a terrible parent. I understood your cruelty. It hurt, still hurts, but I get it."

"I was cruel to *you*? That makes no sense," I said, staring into the clouds. "One little apology can't erase years of abuse. I mean, you pretty much ruined my childhood."

Dad shrugged. "I don't really understand it myself, but this is how it works. I told you this isn't my first rodeo. I've apologized to hundreds of souls...my parents, friends, bosses, social workers, parole officers, people I stole from, people I didn't even know."

"Every time I do it, I get closer to something...good. Call it God, Valhalla, Nirvana, Candyland, somewhere over the rainbow, hell, I don't know, but when I apologize, it's real and I feel better. You're the last one, Adam."

"Well, that's just swell," I said with a thick side of sarcasm. "I die and somehow, it's my job to make you feel better?"

Without missing a beat, he ignored my outrage, and he asked me, "What's the *best* memory you have of me?"

The question conjured a whisper of an image: Dad, dressed in my mom's leopard-print bathrobe with a black shower cap on his head. He had clownishly applied lipstick and rouge to his face. He was carrying a purse and his hairy legs ended in a pair of bright orange fuzzy slippers.

As if he had read my mind, Dad let out a cackling laugh I hadn't heard since childhood and said, "Oh, that? Really?" It was a giggly, high-pitched noise and it startled me at first, but it made me smile. When I looked into his eyes, I saw him, not as a hated-alcoholic-abusive-motherfucker, but as a pleasant old gray-haired guy, lounging comfortably in his Adirondack chair.

"It just popped into my head. I remember laughing and feeling safe," I said.

"But you don't recall anything about why I was dressed like that?"

I had only the image, not the context. "No" I replied.

So, with great alacrity, he told the story:

"It was before your mom committed suicide." He added this detail without a trace of remorse and continued. "You must've been three, maybe four years old and your mom was working late at the hospital cafeteria. Anyway, you started bawling for your mother and you wouldn't stop. "

"Every time I tried to console you, you screamed louder. I was afraid the neighbors might call the cops! Then, I had this idea: Maybe, if I could make you laugh, you'd stop crying."

As he recounted the situation, I flashed to images of his feet scurrying back and forth, as I hid, wailing, under his and my mother's bed.

"I went to the bathroom, grabbed your mother's robe and put it on. I smeared her lipstick and rouge on my lips and cheeks and put her shower cap on my head. I slid into her fuzzy bedroom slippers and, as a finishing touch to my ensemble, I clutched her fancy sequined purse to my chest.

Then, in the highest register I could achieve, I chirped, *"Where's Mama's little man?"*

I was somehow feeling his words as the images flashed clearly through my memory. When I saw the fuzzy slippers at the end of his hairy legs, I did in fact stop crying and ventured a furtive glance, poking my teary face just beyond the bedspread. In a single breath I went from crying to laughing.

"Come give your precious Mama a hug, honey!"

Quickly, playfully, I tucked myself back under the bed. "You're not my mother," I said, trying to frown but it was no use. His daddy-mama routine had broken my tantrum.

"Well, I am, too," he chirped emphatically. *"If I weren't your mother, how would I know where the ice cream is hidden?"* Of course, I never believed for a second that he was my mother, but when he conjured the specter of that ice cream in the freezer, I decided to play along with the deception. After that, the memories became clear: Scooting out from under the bed, a piggyback ride to the kitchen, sitting on the counter while he dished up two big bowls of vanilla with Hershey's syrup glugged on top.

He read Peter Rabbit to me. We watched Sesame Street. We played hide and seek, him still wearing lipstick and my mother's robe. The last thing I remember was waking up to my mother's kiss and my dad, still in costume, passed out drunk on the sofa, beside me.

The next day, she packed my He-Man suitcase, set me on the front porch and told me to wait for a woman in a blue car. Then, Mommy took an overdose of Valium. The lady in the blue car took me to her house and at some point (I really can't say how long) Dad came to get me. All he ever told me was that mom had gone to Heaven and she was very sorry she had to leave.

"Where's Mom now?" My own voice sounded childish, like a whisper of words that should never be spoken.

"She's around," he said causally, as if she'd just gone out the back door. 'We'll get to her later." As almost an afterthought, he added, "You never once blamed her for leaving you. Innately, you seemed to understand that her leaving was in response to me, not you. You found a sense of righteousness in reserving all the hate and blame for me. We're going to need to deal with that first."

Six months after the suicide, neighbors started noticing I was looking scrawny and unkempt. That's when Social Services started keeping a half-assed eye on Dad. For a few years he was a 'functioning' alcoholic. He managed to hold down a job, for the most part. He kept me fed and mostly in school, but the truth is, I took care of him as much as he took care of me. I knew I was a child and that I needed him. That dependency just made me hate him even more.

Ultimately, our symbiosis turned parasitic. I was missing school, selling stuff from the house to buy milk, groceries. Sometimes, I would steal a pack of mac and cheese from the Magic Mart, but I never got caught.

I was eventually placed with a couple of older foster parents. With kindness and thousands of dollars in therapy, they gave me the love every child deserves. Even so, the sins of my father had left deep scars.

Sitting next to him in the Adirondack chair, I got lost in a tangle of memories, some buried so deeply, they only registered as shadows, flashbacks to scenes of abuse, neglect and shame, but also lighter moments. Snippets of smiles and laughter. It was once again Dad's voice that hauled me back.

"Let me help you out here, Sport," he said. "What your soul is coming to terms with is the delusion of judgement, specifically your judgement of me. These are delusions you've carefully curated into a fortress of righteous indignation. You're still hanging on to the notion that, if you can see me miserable and consumed with guilt, that it will somehow make you happy. If I have learned anything in death," he continued, "it's that peace in one's soul is never built on the pain and suffering of others. Counterintuitive as it may seem, seeing me suffer won't make you feel better."

When I didn't disagree with him, he continued.

"Allow me to show you a short cut to the terminus of Memory Lane: Why is it that you never hated your mother for committing suicide?"

"That's easy," I said quickly and honestly. "It wasn't her fault. I believe she thought it was her only escape from you. I cannot, will not, forgive you for that."

I had imagined this moment countless times: The grand finale of my anger, the last, crushing blow that would have him begging my forgiveness. Instead, it was a matter-of-fact declaration, spoken in measured tones.

"Neither your hate nor your forgiveness will have any impact on me," Dad said with a shrug. "The only way *you're* going to feel better is to ask for *my* forgiveness. Then, maybe you can offer both of us the same grace you invented for your mother."

At first, I didn't think I had heard him right. "That's the second time you've implied I should ask you to forgive me!"

"Yep. Oh, I'm not saying I wasn't an alcoholic-asshole-dad. I was. Alcohol retarded and blocked my emotional development. I never grew up, and for that, I am sorry. But you! You've been schlepping around with that chip on your shoulder since childhood. The bigger you got, the bigger it got. Now that you're dead and I'm dead, it's just taking up space in your soul, son. Let it go. It's only causing pain and isolation for you, not me."

Somehow, I had forgotten it was my dad talking. The phrase, "terminus of Memory Lane" resonated, almost poetically. It conjured the image of a great wall at the end of a road to nowhere. In that instant, the clouds surrounding us morphed into a circular gray brick wall. It was as if we were sitting at the bottom of a deep well."

"Nobody gets out until you give in," Dad said with a sigh.

Upon closer study of the bricks in the well, I was able to make out messages. Some were only a single word. Others strung together in long sentences, paragraphs even. I realized each brick held a memory or a snippet from my past. They were stories of anger, sadness, abandonment, fear, loneliness, shame…a veritable carnival side show of misery that I'd built over a lifetime of…rage?

I walked around, reading them. At some point, I even pulled my big chair closer to the wall, intermittently standing in it and scooting it along as I read and remembered everything.

I stood, precariously in the chair to keep reading above my eye level and far as I could go. The stories were all different, yet the message led to the obvious conclusion: My greedy need to hate had finally closed in on me and this was my last chance at grace. This was the dead end of Memory Lane and the only way out led through some kind of forgiveness gate.

"Ok, I get the not-to-subtle message, Dad. I am a prisoner of my own hatred, right? And all I need to do is let you forgive me and we're off to Kum-by-yah?"

"Almost. It's not just about me forgiving you and you forgiving me. It's about me forgiving you and then," he paused with a sly grin and dramatic flair, "it's about you forgiving yourself."

"You keep saying that, but I don't understand. What did I do?" I shouted. "I was a child! The victim! It's a freaking miracle I turned out ok! Know what? I was relieved when I heard you'd died. Finally, you were out of my life! But now, here I am, dead and you're still here!"

"Aye, there's the rub, Hamlet," Dad said as he hopped up out of his chair and began to pace. He was almost dancing!

"Here you are, dead with me and here we'll be until you ask forgiveness. Adam, what if I had cancer, ALS or dementia? Would you have expected me to be a good dad? What if I had been a crappy father because of schizophrenia? Paranoia? Psychosis? As an adult, could you have maybe found a shred of compassion for *me*?"

"Maybe, but that's beside the point. Are you going to tell me now that all your dereliction as a father was beyond your control? That the *devil* made you do it?"

"In a manner of speaking, yes," he said calmly, exhaustedly, as if he'd reach the end of a guessing game

116

with a very dull partner. I'd finally hit upon the right answer.

"My devil was addiction and I loved her," he said it with passion and regret. "She was always there and was she ever devoted! After your mother killed herself, I tried to straighten out. I went to AA but the memory of your mother, even you, were no match for my love of booze.

"The way I saw it then, you were the only thing standing between me and my next drunken stupor. So, I let you go. Social services took you away the morning after the night I spent in jail on that DUI arrest. They found you a nice home and, except for all that hate you've been carrying around, you turned out ok. You were able to find purpose in your life. You're a good doctor. You have compassion for all. Except me.

"But, once you grew up, you never asked, why. 'Why did my dad become an abusive drunk?' You easily forgave your mother for committing suicide. You found empathy for her."

"Because I understood her pain," I blurted out in anger. "It was the surest way she could find to get away from you!"

"But Adam," he said softly, "Didn't you ever wonder how the same guy who dressed up in drag and read Peter Rabbit could also slap your face, in front of all your friends, on the free throw line? I had a disease, Adam, a chemically induced infection of the brain known as alcoholism. I'm sorry I didn't get help. I'm sorry I abused you, but what about what you did to me? My sins were fueled by addiction. Yours were intentional and deliberately cruel. I stayed out of your life for all those years. I'd get sober for a while, but never enough to trust myself around you for long. You finished high school. When I asked to come to your graduation, you didn't even return my call. You blocked my number every time I got a new phone."

"I showed up once in the ER, dehydrated and badly malnourished. I asked for you, my son the doctor. I heard you tell the EMT I wasn't your father and I heard you walk away."

I just sat there, angry at the false equivalency of his argument and at the same time, ashamed that everything he'd just said was true.

"Adam, forgiveness is the only true charity. It's easy to give and forgive when one is rich in compassion. Your whole life, you've been a veritable philanthropist in forgiveness...except for me. Righteous indignation has been your disease. For all of it, I forgive you. Now, to find peace, all you need to do is forgive me and forgive yourself."

And with that, he was gone. Like some kind of evangelical hologram, his image disintegrated without so much as a whisper.

Silently, the gray bricks around me evaporated into a mist. Once again, I was back in the clouds, but the Adirondack chairs were gone and I was standing in front of a flat gray wall, the terminus of Memory Lane. Slowly, the wall became slightly shiny. It was a frosted, sliding glass door! In the distance behind the glass, I could hear footsteps and see a figure walking toward me. The doors swooshed open and there stood my mother, dressed in scrubs and a lunch-lady hair net.

She smiled and said, "Hey, Dr. Adam. There's a guy in here wearing a woman's bathrobe, a shower cap and fuzzy orange slippers. He said to tell you he knows where the ice cream is."

What was left of my icy rage melted, welling into tears. If she could forgive him, so could I and, if I could forgive him, maybe he could forgive me? The hatred and indignation I had nurtured for so long vanished into a swell of forgiveness and gratitude. "That's my dad," I said, smiling as she welcomed me into her into my arms. "I'm his son."

Note from Nancy:

Dr. Adam saw me in the ER once. Nice boy with the sweetest brown eyes. His story confirmed something I'd heard from many in the afterlife: True forgiveness isn't just for the forgiven. Its largesse bestows an afterglow upon the forgiver and leaves redemption all the way around.

Roslyn's Story

I'm not a doctor but I'm pretty sure if you die, (of cancer) the cancer dies at the same time.
-Norm McDonald

Only the good die young.
-Oliver Hereford (and Billy Joel. Ok, we've all said this one!)

I'd been sick my whole life, all 5 years of it. Neuroblastoma was what the doctors said. I named it 'Toma' for short. Toma was the Joker to my Batman. The Voldemort to my Harry Potter and ultimately, I gave my life to kill Toma. At least, that's the way I look at it.

For some time, I was more dead than alive. My disease paralyzed me, metastasized to my spine, liver, lungs. That's what doctors say when they know your cancer starts eating at you in unexpected places. My lungs were where the cancer finally met its match, and I died killing it.

The death of a child is considered tragic, but when you're the kid dying, it's all you've ever known so it seems normal. When our preacher would come to visit, he would always pray with us just before he left. Mostly he prayed for God's will to be done. That, to me was a goofy prayer. Even a 5-year-old knows if God is as all-powerful as everybody says He is, He's going to see to it that He gets His way, without me praying for it.

So, one day, I asked, "But preacher, what if God's plan is for me to die with cancer? What if His will is for me to get sicker and die?" I knew my mom and dad wouldn't like the question. I knew it would put the preacher on the spot, but I asked anyway.

Both the preacher and I looked at my parents, then back at each other. Their faces were masks of grief, weary from sleepless nights that ended with no good news at dawn.

"Nobody knows God's plan," the preacher said with a shrug. "But God likes it when we ask for his help. Let's pray again and this time, you ask God for what you want."

I agreed. I started by asking God to help my parents and to take care of them after I died. I asked God to save my soul and take me to heaven. And I asked God to let me live, in Heaven and become a grownup in Heaven, with kids of my own. The preacher, cried. Mom and Dad cried. I figured it was a pretty good prayer. That was the day before the night I died.

As I left my cancer-riddled body behind, I remember thinking of a line from *Good Night Moon*:

Good night stars
Good night air
Good night noises everywhere!

I truly expected to hear angels singing amid white puffy clouds with silver linings but with the last beat of my heart, I heard a new cadence! A different rhythm emerged. Instead of the "bump-thump, bump-thump" of a heartbeat, I distinctly heard the "tap: rat-a-tat-tat! Tap: rat-a-tat-tat" of a snare drum! It was the little drummer boy from the Christmas song! He motioned to me and said one word: "Come".

He played, marched and I followed. It was the first time in ages my legs had been able to walk by themselves and the first time in my memory that I wasn't in pain. Before long, I was skipping more than walking. In time to the "tap: rat-a-tat-tat," I started singing a song my daddy taught me:

"Here she comes just a-walking down the street
Singing do-wa-diddy -diddy -dum-diddy -de."

I was so into it that I didn't even notice when the drummer boy stopped marching and I bumped right into him!

"Sorry," I said, laughing. "It's been so long since I skipped and sang, I forgot how to stop!"

Drummer boy was not amused. "You have an appointment," he dryly pronounced. "Wait here." And with that, the kid with the drum turned smartly on his heels and skipped off in the direction whence we came.

I turned around and found myself at the end of a long line of other kids. Some were talking to each other. Some were playing games like hopscotch and rock-paper-scissors, but we all seemed to be lined up for something.

"Excuse me," I said to the little girl immediately in front of me. "Why are we in line?"

"I can't say," the little girl replied. "A girl, blowing on a conch shell and shaking little brass bells, brought me here and told me to wait. It was festive! I thought like, maybe we were going to a party. I haven't seen her since."

"A prince riding a lion brought me here," said the kid next in line. "He let me put my face in the lion's mane!"

Before long, a knot of us kids had broken from the line and we were all talking about where we came from, how we were ushered in and what disease or accident had killed us to get here. Nobody was the least bit ashamed or self-conscious about their illness or fearful of scaring the others. We shared stories about our ailments, injuries, surgeries, treatments. We all knew words most children don't, like the names of pain medications and protocols for chemo and immuno-therapies.

We'd all experienced how healthy kids would try to be nice but most just didn't know how. They seemed afraid they might hurt us, say the wrong thing or "catch" what we had. They also didn't want to make friends with someone who was dying. I got that. When I was first diagnosed, I made friends with some of the other cancer kids, but they died, so I just gave up on friends.

Then, there were also the mean kids who made fun of us, laughed at our kid-sized walkers, our thinning hair, or the tubes up our noses. They'd pretend to be nice to our faces and then mock us behind our backs, but we always knew.

But here? We were all just happy to be out of the hospital, out of our beds and unhooked from our IVs. Here, we had glorious mops of hair! We wore clothes and sneakers, not pajamas and bedroom shoes. Here, whatever this place was, we were just kids. Clouds or no clouds, I had no doubt I was in Heaven.

If anyone did question our whereabouts, those doubts were soon to be firmly dashed. My little tribe of children was now sitting cross-legged, in a circle, telling each other about ourselves, asking questions, when a tall, dark teenaged girl approached us. She was older than us kids, but not by much. I'd say she was just about babysitting age.

"Hello, and may I have your attention, please?" She looked and sounded like an Angel. Clearly, her white robe and lilting voice were designed to suspend any belief to the contrary.

Slowly, we children quieted down and stood to face her. When she was certain she had our undivided attention, she broke into a big smile, threw her arms out wide and said, "Welcome to Heaven!"

A few of us clapped. Some bounced up and down in uncontrollable excitement and a few ran into the Angel's waiting arms to be rewarded with a group hug. The exuberance however quickly dissipated. We fell silent again as our new visitor asked for calm and continued.

"I'm a saint, well a martyr, really. My name is Philomena. What you are experiencing is known as the Law of Conservation of Energy. That just means energy can neither be created nor destroyed and that energy can only be transferred or changed from one form to another. You were alive and sick. Now, your physical, earthly energy has been transformed into pure prana, or spiritual energy. Ta-da! Change! Questions? Yes?"

She pointed to a little boy who had furtively raised his hand. Looking down at his sneakers, he quietly mumbled, "I wanna go home."

"I see. And how many are you?" Philomena asked.

The little boy held up four fingers and added, "and a quarter."

"Oh, sweetie," Philomena's eyes teared up a little. "Four and a quarter-years old is the perfect age to want home. I get it. But I think there's something else you all want to do here, even more than going home?"

Philomena looked right at me and said, "and what would you like to do, young lady?"

Remembering the preacher's words, about God wanting us to ask for His help, I knew my question instantly. It slipped out of my mouth fast as I could form the words. With deep conviction and sincerity, I said, "Miss Philomena, may we just play?"

Well, you'd have thought I just announced the circus was coming to town! All the kids, even the whining four and a quarter-year-old longing for home, eagerly whispered, "Yes! Please, may we play a while?"

Philomena said, "Alrighty then, who wants to play?" Even though every hand went into the air, she pretended to count us. Then, she smiled and said, "The players have a majority! Everybody play!"

And that is exactly what we did. It began with games that required only our imaginations: Hide-and-seek. One-Two-Three Red Light, I Spy, Who Am I, Red Rover. We made up riddles and the most ridiculous Knock-Knock jokes we could imagine.

Then, we started playing games and sports we vaguely recalled. From Archery to Zorkhaneh wrestling games, kids from all over the world who had recently died horrible deaths, were kicking balls, wrestling, shuffling cards, throwing dice, skipping ropes and swimming, running, jumping in ways our bodies would have never found possible during our brief and painful earthly existences.

We learned rules to old games and when we tired of old games, we made up new ones. We found that almost anything could be a game! Sometimes we played make-believe, becoming kings and queens, pirates and cowboys, musicians, astronauts and bakers of glorious mud pies. We dug holes to nowhere and then filled them back up again.

Little did we know, we were preparing for yet another adventure, another turn at life.

When they told the preacher that I had died. He silently and simultaneously prayed and cried. He asked God to take my soul (As if God might absentmindedly leave it somewhere!) He prayed that God, in His wisdom, would comfort my parents and help them to know I was happy in God's house. The preacher may not have known much about God or Heaven, but that part of his prayer was answered. I was very happy, even though I knew my death had made my parents sad beyond any suffering I'd ever known.

At first, this bothered me. Again, recalling the preacher's words, I asked God why my death made me so happy and my parents so sad.

"I hear you've got questions?" It was Philomena. "Well, I've got one for you: Do you know what a prism is?" She asked.

"It's that glass thing that makes rainbows?" I ventured.

"That's a good definition," Philomena said smiling. "It takes light in and refracts it into all the different colors of the spectrum. Same white light, just split up to look different. In death, it's as if your soul has passed through a prism. The people who loved you can only see and remember what you were like on earth. They can't see all the potential you have and will experience here, in Heaven. Therefore, they are sad, but you, like light through a prism, have been transformed. You're experiencing all the colors,

so to speak, playing, learning and happy as a little clam."
She put her hand in mine and indicated we should take a
'closed walk'. I had no idea what that meant, but I knew
Philomena was great at telling stories and I wanted to suck
up every word like a big fat sponge.

"When a person dies, it is never random," she
said. "Certain souls are selected to go through experiences,
to be developed in iterations. It's called reincarnation.
Others are born and live out their existence in much longer
lives, never to be repeated.

"But when it comes to children, the repeats are special.
The children who suffered illness on earth? Their souls
absorb powerful neurophysical responses during their
short, sickly lives. Many of you see your parents,
hopelessly suffer the emotional, physical and often
financial pain of your fate. Some kids lived completely
abandoned in cultures where a mortally deformed or
defective child is viewed as a stain on the family. Yet, for all
your stoic wisdom, your lives sorely lacked that most
fundamental occupation of childhood: In life, you rarely
got to play.

"In your brief lives, you felt the love, anguish, the pity,
patience and gratitude of those who saw you as 'not long
for this world.' You endured pain and indignity, often
without understanding why. You learned to exist, without

assigning blame, goodness or evil, to your circumstances. Yet, for all your suffering, you didn't get to 'test drive' life."

"But here, in Heaven, it's different?" I asked with a smile and a skip.

"Oh, you think so?" Said Philomena and she made a funny face.

"Yep!" I said, with a little dance. "Here, in Heaven, all we do is play! We solve problems, we make believe and create! Our souls and imaginations know no bounds. As far as I can tell, there is no such thing as failure, only infinite ideas and possibilities. Bad luck simply doesn't exist! If a concept or a game doesn't work, we just tweak it or move on to something new. Everything we do here is fun, and everything leads us to something better."

I had many such conversations with Philomena, but most of my time was spent playing with the other kids. Every game, fantasy and experiment taught us, built our knowledge or sent us chasing something completely new. Nothing was impossible!

What started as simple, childhood games, evolved into an unshakable belief that we were being led by an energy, a power that would always bring our efforts to an inevitable truth.

In play, we collaborated, we swapped costumes, built on each other's stories. We breathlessly exchanged make-believe flights of fancy. That original, desperate wish to "just play" became the gateway to our next reality.

I have no clue how long this evolution went on. Hours? Eons? There was simply no beginning or end to the fun of playing, inquiring, sharing and learning. It was as if every fiber of our beings was sopping up faith in some yet to be explained super-collider of knowledge.

Gradually, we evolved from games and riddles to imagining new possibilities in science and nature. We concocted intricate math theories and laughed like little hyenas when they disintegrated into absurdity.

We thought the most outrageous, crazy ideas and put them into stories, paintings and beautiful songs. We built imaginary cities. We mulled over ways to cure our own diseases! Our play morphed into concepts that, one day, might be considered miracles of sheer genius.

Philomena was often walking among us as we played. New kids would arrive, and familiar faces would disappear, but Philomena was a constant, always nearby, smiling, always ready to answer questions and join the discourse.

There was a group of us, standing before a blackboard, discussing quantum mechanics. A little boy, wearing a baseball cap backwards, a kimono and a holstered toy six gun, emphatically said, "I'm telling you; quantum electromagnetism is basically the foundation of almost everything."

To which I replied, "Basically? Almost? You call that a theorem? You are such a baby!" And several of us threw our chalk at him. He laughed and threw a few pieces back.

Philomena just watched and as the others wandered away, she touched my arm and said, "Walk with me."

"Open walk, or closed?" I asked, slyly and Philomena laughed. I'd learned so much since our first conversation about light and prisms. It was a very nerdy way of asking whether we were going to a place of no return or coming back.

"You have learned a lot, young lady," Philomena said as we strolled along. "This will be an open walk."

The notion of an open walk thrilled and excited me. You see, in graph theory, an open walk is said to have different starting and ending vertices, i.e., the origin vertex and terminal vertex are different. A "closed" walk, however, starts and ends at the same vertex, like a loop. Wherever we were going, Philomena was telling me, I wasn't coming back.

"In life," Philomena began, "you learned the limits of your body. Most people don't do that until they're quite old, but your body was challenged from the get-go. You died knowing there was much more to life than physical autonomy and here, "she gestured broadly at our surroundings, "this is where you learned that play is the gateway to intellect and intellect is an "open walk" into the Mind of God."

"Is that where we are now?" I whispered in awe-inspired reverence, "inside the Mind of God?"

"Gosh, no!" Laughed Philomena, "even I haven't seen the Mind of God! Don't know anyone who has. It was just a figure of speech. Remember our conversation about the prism? Your time here has helped you see the light, break it into components, scramble it and reassemble the colors in infinite ways. You're ready for another shot at earthly existence. Everything in your first life and the playtime in Heaven has teed you up for another trip back through the prism."

"But I'm so happy here," I said as we ambled along. "Come to think of it, I don't even recall what it was like on earth!"

"And you won't remember. In fact, you won't remember playing in Heaven either, but as you grow and learn and play on earth, you will automatically grasp concepts that others find difficult. You will 'split the light,' see and understand patterns long before your peers. You won't remember Heaven, but you will…," she thought for a moment before saying, "…embody it.

In your next life, you and the others like you will be the geniuses, the artists, scientists and deep thinkers who challenge everything. You will solve the world's famines and droughts, eradicate illness, discover great sources of energy. You will design, invent, build and tear down with wisdom even you will not understand."

"Will I remember you?" I asked. "Will I even know we were ever here?"

Philomena shook her head, but she was smiling. "No, not even a whisper of a memory. There will be times when you have a feeling of recognition, a glint of an idea that maybe you have experienced or read something before, but it will flit by, and you'll get right back to your important work. In your next life, you'll play, work and grow. You will have the satisfaction of making your parents so proud of you."

"But what about my first parents, the ones who buried me. Are they going to be ok?"

Philomena took me in her arms and said, "Your compassion is strong, little one. And yes, they are ok. Their greatest grief was not in losing you so young, but in being robbed of the future they imagined for you. Never in their wildest dreams could they have envisioned what you will achieve."

As we ended our embrace, I heard a faint but growing "thump-bumping" coming our way. Sure enough, my drummer boy was back, but this time he wasn't tapping on a little snare drum. Instead, he was bumping out a deep beat on a sonorous, no-nonsense bass drum. I was quite sure it was to be my new heartbeat.

And suddenly, as quickly as I had died, the soul of that pitifully sick kid was born again. Imbued with health, strength and the joys of play, I was off on an earnest quest to explore, to be led in an open walk, into the very Mind of God, metaphorically speaking.

Note from Nancy:

I spoke to a few children using the Hooligan, but little Ros's story was the most coherent. I swear, some of those little souls were too rambunctious to be bothered! She had been the great-granddaughter of one of the residents at my nursing home. Honestly, I don't recall ever meeting her, but she remembered me and that's how we got to talking on the Hooligan.

Her story was the most disturbing and yet the most thought-provoking I've heard in my adventures. Like most of you, I could never figure out why a loving, omnipotent God would visit pain and suffering on the least of us.

After hearing what Roslyn had to say, the phrase, "suffer the little children to come unto Me," took on a richer meaning. It's not just about children being worthy of grace. Suffering isn't the end game. It's their very suffering that helps them eagerly accept Heaven's unlimited grace for themselves and in the next life, they liberally break it down, like the light through a prism, and return to share it with the world.

What it took me much longer to appreciate was the crossroads where the Law of Conservation of Energy, light of a prism and the concepts of open and closed walks in graph theory all intersect. I'm no whiz when it comes to math and physics, but somewhere in that sop of space-time and energy, I stumbled upon the concept of 'time geography.'

There's a case to be made that life, in every form, whether physical or metaphysical, exists on an incomprehensible and infinite playing field of space and time, light and dark, matter and antimatter. All the life paths become captured within this net of constraints and contradictions, some of which are imposed by the physiology of human bodies and the laws of earthly physics.

But there are planes within the universe where these laws don't necessarily apply. These planes exist outside the so-called net of constraints and contradictions. Maybe this is the area where energy, light and infinite open walks converge to reveal the Mind of God? I have no proof, but to me, it explains genius and everything little Ros told me. And it makes a whole lot more sense than most of the rigmarole one reads in the Book of Revelation!

Maggie's Story

Everything you can imagine is real.

-Pablo Picasso

*Faith is to believe what you do not see; the reward of
this faith is to see what you believe."*

-St. Augustine

The day I died had been such a beautiful day. It was early summer, about an hour shy of sunset. Still warm but with the gentle breezes that often accompany dusk this time of year. I was coming back from the grocery store where I'd bought all the stuff to make cucumber pickles that evening.

Now, I recall hearing some soldiers say they heard the bullet that hit them, but I didn't hear a thing. Even the marksman who shot me didn't know until days later what had happened. It was an accident, of course. Hell, if he'd been trying to hit me, me driving a car at 60mph and him 100 yards away, he'd most likely've missed.

I was one of those Christians who believed getting to Heaven was going to be quite a production. The way my preachers told it, Jesus was coming back for us believers. The dead would be waiting patiently in our graves and the living believers would be going about our business and instantly disappear in the Rapture!

Personally, I loved the notion of everyone in the world, just living life, when suddenly, all the Christian believers evaporate! Sometimes, when I couldn't sleep, I'd imagine how the media and the politicians would explain that! 'We interrupt this program to bring you an important message: All who believed in the resurrection of Jesus have vanished. Pilots in mid-air, construction workers, teachers, surgeons, gone! Christian cemeteries and graveyards lay riddled with holes and broken caskets! Details at eleven!'

That's exactly what I *thought* had happened when I got shot! I figured my soul had an express ticket, straight from that old Pontiac Bonneville into a glorious parade, dancing into Heaven to a rousing rendition of 'When the Saints Go Marching In."

Only, it didn't happen like that at all.

Instead of being caught up in a festive, ostentatious procession of freshly harvested souls, I was standing alone in what appeared to be a lush garden, awash in every shade of green you could imagine, speckled with a kaleidoscope of fragrant flowers.

I was beginning to grasp the fact that I was dead and probably in the Garden of Eden when a trumpet sounded in the distance, and I heard a voice. A man, emerged from the bramble, singing.

"I come to the garden alone, while the dew is still on the roses." I knew the hymn and I finished the verse,

"And the voice I hear, falling on my ear, the Son of God dis-clooooooses." In life, I wasn't much of a singer and apparently, that hadn't been remedied in death. I still couldn't carry a tune in a bucket with a lid on it.

"That was awful," my new acquaintance laughed. "All God's children have gifts, but a singing voice isn't one of yours. I'm Jesus Christ."

He continued to walk toward me, opened his arms and gave me a big hug. It was about that time I noticed we were both wearing silky white robes and...glowing, ever so slightly.

"You look just as I imagined," I whispered with genuine enthusiasm. He was about my height (5'7") slender and dark with brown hair and brown eyes.

140

I had long ago given up the idea that Jesus was a white man. I mean, there were no blonde, blue eyed Jews running around Jerusalem back in the day. No, this guy was the real deal, and I was delighted to met him.

"And do you know why I look just like you expected?" Jesus said with a mischievous grin.

"Because you believed! You imagined, you had faith in a Heaven where you would get a new body, where you'd see Me. You believed I would prepare a place for you and all the other true believers. Well done, o' good and faithful servant," he said as he clapped me on the back, punctuating his praise. As you might imagine, I was literally tickled to death!

There we were, all smiling and glowing when Jesus said, "Heaven is as you imagined it *because* you imagined! It was all in your head, girl. What you're experiencing in death is exactly what you expected it to be because you imagined it this way."

"But I imagined the Rapture! What happened to that?"

"Nothing," said Jesus with a shrug. "It just hasn't happened yet. You have some vivid beliefs about the Rapture, but you don't know the Rapture or Hell, for that matter, like you know me," Jesus replied. "God will lift the veil on the Rapture, Heaven and Hell when the time comes. For now, just abide in me."

This puzzled me. My mind raced to reconcile the nuances between belief, make-believe, imagination and faith. If Jesus was created in my imagination, what about all the horrible things I'd imagined and believed about Hell?

As if reading my thoughts, Jesus said, "Oh, don't worry 'bout that! Hell is but a shadow, an ill- formed thought that will soon dissolve entirely from your memory."

"Then, there's no Hell?" I gasp in disbelief.

"Not for you. Let me put it this way: Your imagination is the most beautiful, sacred, holy part of your existence. It is a human being's superpower. You went to church. You read your Bible. Your brain made indelible images of what I looked like, what Heaven looks like. Those imaginings became like memories. It is why you can 'remember' me as clearly as you remember your own mother.

Before I could express my next thought, Jesus said, "And yes, this applies to everyone, not just those who believe in Me. The bonds between imagination and faith are incontrovertible, immutable and nonnegotiable. For you," Jesus continued, "there is no Hell because you never imagined *me* there. And, since you couldn't imagine yourself anywhere in death without me, Hell, for you simply could not exist. Make sense?"

When I didn't immediately respond, Jesus said, "walk with me," and we set out together, strolling through the garden.

As we walked, I saw others, clothed exactly as Jesus and me, softly glowing. Drawing closer to my fellow Paradisians, (what else would you call someone living in paradise) I began to see other similarities. They were all the same size, shape, skin tone. Everyone was wearing the silky white robe, and they all had that same style hair. They all had that golden aura, just like Jesus and me.

In fact, on closer scrutiny, I realized they ALL looked exactly like Jesus! How to broach this with the 'Jesus' standing next to me? This, I most certainly had not imagined, at least not in this particular configuration!

As we continued to walk in silence, I sidled over to the edge of a nearby pond, with the intent of stealing a glance at my own reflection. Sure enough, instead of Maggie Jones, 68, from White Stone, South Carolina, the image in the water was none other than my Lord and Savior, Jesus Christ.

"Ah, Jesus…," saying His name felt like I was starting a prayer, "is it my imagination or does everyone here look like you?"

He seemed genuinely pleased that I'd noticed. "Yes, it's your imagination and, yes, everyone here looks like me

143

because all of you *are* me! We're all truly one in 'the body of Christ.'"

For the longest time, I stared at my reflection, then at Jesus, then back at my reflection, then at all the other Jesuses, milling around the garden. They all seemed to be engaged in animated chatter, sometimes laughing, other times gravely serious in their discussions. A few of the Jesuses were alone, staring off into space or just sitting, meditating with eyes closed.

"This is another one of those things you know, but you were missing the context to fully understand," he chuckled. "You know God is omnipresent. You interpreted that to mean God's 'presence' is everywhere. What you failed to fully imagine is how this might be achieved. Well, this is how God achieves omnipresence in Heaven. You, Me, all who have died, become a part of God. In your case, reborn in Jesus, *as Jesus*. Jesus continued, "We all look alike here because in God's eyes, our souls are all the same. We are all God's creation."

Again, I nodded, but still had no idea where this was going.

"Like most of God's mysteries, the answer is there if you look for it," Jesus said as we continued our walk.

"This little puzzle was solved for you in Second Corinthians, 3:16-18: 'But, whenever someone turns to the Lord, the veil is taken away...So all of us who have had that veil removed can see and reflect the glory of the Lord. And the Lord—who is the Spirit—makes us more and more like Jesus and we are changed into *his glorious image*."

"No one comes to the Father except through me." I mumbled, reciting from John, 14:6 from memory.

"Exactly", said Jesus. "And in John's way of thinking, getting through me, for Christians, involves becoming me, at least for a while. Just think about it. Pray on it."

Jesus patted my shoulder. His touch felt warm, soft and comforting as I did indeed reflect on my inevitable, spiritual journey, imagining a totally heretofore unimaginable way of living in Christ, as Christ.

I'd known Miss Nancy since I was born. It wasn't until I started volunteering at her Senior Living facility that I learned she could talk to the dead. Not that I believed a word of it, but I did believe that *she* believed it, so I just listened when she'd bring me up to date on her latest chit-chats with residents of the hereafter.

I'd heard everything about our friends Betty, and poor Gavin, and even the ones I didn't know, like little Roslyn, Dr. Adam, Frankie and Leon. The notion that different people had different afterlives was just nonsense to me, but the way Nancy told her tales, was entertaining.

Now, here I was, dead, having Jesus himself tell me Miss Nancy was right! I was keen on calling her and hoping the Hooligan really worked. Thank Jesus, it did!

Nancy's the one who told me how I'd died. Seems the Sprague boys were target shooting with a new long-range rifle. The newspaper called it an X-Bolt Hell's Cannon! What a name! The single shot went right through my head, in the left temple, out the right. I didn't go through Hell, but ironically, the Hell's Cannon sent a bullet right through me!

I was dead before my car bumped the side of the post office and bounced into Joe Pierce's Garden. The post office was barely damaged but about half of Joe's corn and several tomato plants were plowed up under the car. The news story quoted him lamenting my death, but saying it was, "fortunately early enough in the season to replant". Life goes on.

I told Nancy about all the Jesus clones and how I was a Jesus clone, too. She laughed and asked me to try walking on water!

"Have you ever heard of such a thing?" I asked.

"No, but I'm not surprised. Seems like God just gives us what we need when we die. Maybe what you needed was a little time with Jesus," she added. "Heck, maybe He multiplied all the Jesuses and made you a Jesus, just to speed up the process. Like an immersion class!" Nancy

146

always had clever ways of looking at things. We reminisced a little about our small town and the folks who lived there. I talked mostly about being surprised, and just a tad disappointed, there was no Rapture.

"It's probably like your Jesus said. It might still be coming, just not now," Nancy mused encouragingly. "You just never know what the Almighty's up to."

I supposed she was right. I mean, if someone had tried to tell me that I would die from a bullet, shot out of an X-Bolt Hell's Cannon and find myself in a gaggle of Jesuses, I would have laughed my ass off at the sheer novelty of the story! So far, my death had been way more exciting than my life.

My time on earth had been what most folks would call mundane. I spent most of it not a mile from where I was born. I never longed for or wanted anything I couldn't have. My first and only job was as the secretary at the elementary school, the one where Nancy's wife was the principal. When she died, I figured it was as good a time as any to retire, even though I was only 62.

I was what folks used to call an "old maid" and I didn't find the term offensive. I was old and technically a maiden, so the shoe fit. I was an only child. I lived with my parents and took care of them 'til they died and then, I stayed on in their house. I loved a lot of people, but I never met "the one" and that was just fine.

Going to church, reading, needlepoint, volunteering and putting up pickles and preserves in the summer were my ways of keeping busy in retirement. I figured I'd sell the house and end up at the Senior Living Center with Nancy and that crowd when I couldn't do for myself any longer. But God and the X-Bolt Hell's Cannon had other ideas.

The static on the Hooligan was turning into a roar. I remember hearing Nancy say, "I love you, Maggie. Now go in peace to love and serve your Lord…or yourself, if it turns out you're Jesus!" And with those words, I was back in the afterlife, still glowing and just staring at my Jesus-face, reflected in the pond.

As if he'd been right in middle of my confab with Nancy, Jesus-my-greeter said, "Don't be worried about the Rapture. It'll happen, just not yet. When God's ready, it will all be set in motion and we'll all go to meet God, in glory. Meantime, would you like for me to explain what's going on here?"

I nodded that I would, and Greeter-Jesus began the most fantastic story I'd ever heard.

"Humans have existed for about 300,000 years," Jesus began. "As they watched their young being born and their old die, they began to make up stories that could explain these comings and goings. At first, nobody believed these imaginings. It was more entertainment than dogma.

As centuries passed and humans became more sophisticated, so evolved their stories, imaginings of unseen forces ruling their earthly lives. At first, they intermittently worshipped and cursed the elements, earth, wind, water and fire, as if they were gods. Good spirits helped. Evil spirits harmed.

Cultures grew and so did humanity's collective image of the divine forces guiding their lives. Most of these vague beliefs and later monotheistic faiths painted the deity as a warrior-God, full of wrath and punishment for anyone who didn't toe the line.

This was the whole 'eye-for-an-eye' era, when God (or the gods, depending your brand of religion) smote people on a whim. Yahweh/Allah presumably sanctioned jihads with promises of great riches for martyrdom.

People began to travel and explore. They encountered different faiths, confronted moral differences and similarities in their beliefs. This expansion of physical horizons naturally sparked an expansion of imagination and, in turn spiritual energy. It stoked a notion of a higher purpose, a transcendent moral order.

Living in an interconnected world meant learning to tolerate and accept, even homogenize differences. In order to coexist, humanity began to preach, if not always follow, a 'love-thy-neighbor' image of God."

Wait!" The word popped out of me like a champagne cork. "Are you saying humans invented God?"

"No, honey! I'm saying that God, the Force behind all that is seen and unseen, is slowly and methodically being revealed, down through the millennia, through the human imagination! It is your spiritual tether to this life and what lies beyond. God hasn't changed. Doesn't change. It's human understanding of God that's expanding. The evolution of your physical bodies as well as your human morality and spirituality grow with each generation. Sometimes, in individual spurts, sometimes in massive cultural upheavals."

"And one of those upheavals was Your time on earth, when God sent you, as Jesus, the Christ?" I said this with a sense of uncertainty, not sure I was prepared for the answer.

Jesus shook his head, no. "The truth is, I've never existed anywhere but, in your heart, and mind. Intellectually, you know there's not a shred of evidence I ever walked the earth. Not a single artifact, neither a census record, nor any record of my birth or death."

And then, as if distracted by another thought, Jesus said, "and you can forget right now about all the Holy Wars, the transactional ideas of churches, priests, faiths healers and messiahs! The pieces of the cross that were bought and sold? The Shroud of Turin? All phonies. All the circumstantial evidence of my life, ministry and death, started to be 'collected' decades after my storied resurrection."

"And yet," I observed, "here we are, chatting away in Heaven." I said as I watched four Jesuses finish up a bocce ball game on the other side of the pond.

"Yep, here we are!" Said Jesus. "What your mind, your spirit, your soul is coming to terms with now is what God ultimately has in store for all Mankind. The infinite nature of God is being revealed to you, through Me, in a way you can process, based on your previous understanding and faith. This experience is different for everyone who leaves their earthly body and enters this next existence, with God.

My mind, my soul were racing. "You mean to tell me that *every* life has an *afterlife* that is unique, and that God is so *omniscient*, all those lives can be accommodated within God?"

"That is a major leap of faith you just made and yes, that's exactly what I am saying. As you abide here, in Heaven, even more will be revealed. When you took communion in church, you imagined, believed, that the bread and wine were a symbol of Me becoming part of you. Now, in death, you have become part of Me! As part of Me, you will continue your path to God's presence. You will continue to evolve morally and spiritually. And through us, Humanity will slowly continue to grow in compassion and grace."

"How?" Sometimes, the simple questions yield the most profound answers.

"That's what we're here to find out, together." Jesus said. "But here's what I do know: Those individual spurts and cultural upheavals of God's revelations, bring us, our eternal souls, ever closer to a peace and love we cannot yet imagine.

"The Rapture, maybe?" I asked.

"Maybe. Or it could be that God is also growing and evolving, too. We may never catch up, but we will continue in God's wake, toward purity and communion."

Suddenly, I was reminded of Dr. Martin Luther King's notion, of judging people by their character and not by outward appearances. Jesus finished my thought with, "...and someday, maybe we can look forward to a world where we don't feel the need to judge each other...at all."

Note from Nancy:

When Maggie told me this last bit, the Hooligan quit working. Just dried up and cut off, as if maybe she'd spilled some Heavenly beans that should've stayed in the jar!

Oh, I still get the occasional little bit of static and even a quick howdy from a soul I've known, but for now, it's mostly quiet. If I get any new information, I'll let you know.

Departing Thoughts

…neither death nor life, neither angels nor demons,
neither the present nor the future, nor any powers,
neither height nor depth, nor anything else in all
creation, will be able to separate us from the love of
God…

-Romans 8:35-39

Imagine there's no heaven. It's easy if you try.

-John Lennon

First off, I'm not dead yet! Just wanted to be sure you understand that I'm writing this for myself and not as a "Hooligan" story from the great beyond.

Before writing "The End," I just need to pass along a few observations I've made in my encounters with the dead. You may want to jot these down somewhere or, if you actually own this book, go ahead and underline a few of these little gems.

At this point, I'm pretty sure the line between living and dead is not a bright one. True, one can't be a little bit dead, but there seem to be at least some spirits who work, unseen, among the living. Still, according to my sources, most of us exit this life, into another one, and (happily) never return.

Understand that in the great, teeming swell of the recently human, my experience is minuscule. Everyone ever contacted through the Hooligan was an acquaintance of mine, or Bertie's or Sean Hooligan's. When you think of all the people on earth who die (about 150,000 a day) and multiply that by weeks, months, years, you begin to see that my little visits with the dead are probably not universally representative. In fact, I'd venture to propose that there are infinite possibilities for what life after death might be.

Maybe I should travel more? I'd love to chat with the soul of an Australian Aboriginal, or a dead Chinese factory worker. I also think about those who have lived marginal lives, the homeless, refugees, the enslaved, the hundreds of thousands who are living right now, tortured by war: how death must be a welcomed release from their torment.

I can just imagine the relief they must feel to know they will never be exhausted, thirsty or hungry again. I well up with tears, when I think of how, in death, they can rest in peace, without the fear of thieves stealing their stuff as they sleep. How in death, they will shake off their constant struggle for survival, the threat of diseases and pain. They will remove their tribulations like filthy old clothes and be washed clean, swaddled in comfort and joy. But then again, that's *my* imagination, *my* connection to God, the Almighty, the Universe.

Which leads me to conclude with the following 'top ten list' of things I have learned from death and about it.

10.   Religion is man-made, but Heaven is real! I take issue with John Lennon. It is *not* easy to imagine there's no Heaven! We simply cannot do it. Now, maybe "Mr.-King-of-the-Liverpool-Fab-Four' was somehow able to imagine no Heaven because, after all, he was John Lennon but for most of us, imagining where we go when we die is practically a clandestine hobby! It is hardwired into our psyche. Imagination must be a gift from Heaven. Therefore, Heaven is real because our imaginations undeniably exist. Descartes was onto something. If only he'd taken the time to finish the reasoning: 'I think

therefore, I am,' with, 'and when I am no more, I can yet imagine where I'll be.'

9. There is no one truth, no singular experience of death. We all led unique lives. Why should we expect the next life to be one-size-fits-all? You think all that extravagant numerology and imagery in the Book of Revelation is pointing to a puffy-cloud-city in the sky? Oh, hell no! I don't pretend to know half of what Revelation is trying to communicate, but the message I've gotten from authentically dead people is one of infinite possibilities.

We must be careful, though. For all we know, a bunch of Christians got together, ate some mushrooms, read some scrolls backwards and *voila*, The Book of Revelation! Don't overthink it. From what I have heard through the Hooligan, everything we need to know about Heaven will be explained when we get there, regardless of whether you're a Zen Buddhist, a Holy Roller or an Atheist.

8. Jesus may have been a carpenter, but his daddy was an Engineer! Just look at your hand. Pull your thumb across your palm. Make a fist. Isn't that amazing? Gaze into a starry night sky. Watch a sunrise. I ask you: How can you look at all that and not *imagine* a Higher Power?

The neuroscience of how we form ideas and memories, how we make peace with inconsistencies, is still a mystery.

We are intentional beings. We do things for a reason; therefore, we assume the Universe is also intentional, and we seek to understand what it wants for us. We may never have a satisfactory answer to the question, 'is there a God', at least not until we die.

7. Sophocles said, 'of all the great wonders, none is greater than man. Only for death can he find no cure.' This presumes death is something we might want to cure, to get rid of! Well, do not sign me up for that! If anything, I'm looking forward to what lies ahead.

Death, for most of us, isn't the end. In my experience, many of us have issues we're going to work through after we die. Whether it's coming to terms with our sins, opening up to forgiveness, loving ourselves or seeing old contradictions explained in new ways. Our last exhale is hardly the end of the storyline: It's just the start of a new page, a new chapter, maybe even a whole new book!

6. As far as I can tell, neither Satan nor Hell exists. Now, I make this assertion with the full understanding that I could be wrong. I've just seen no evidence of Hell or the meeting out of any real punishment for so-called sins and wickedness.

Maybe the truly wicked don't get permission to access the Hooligan? Maybe I haven't found any wicked souls in the afterlife because I never knew any truly wicked people in this life? For now, I'm going with the theory that God or whatever force is running the show isn't a vengeful asshole! The universe, it would appear, wants our next life to be one of peace and love, just like the hippies in the sixties were saying. Hedging my bets, I will continue to lead a godly, righteous and sober life, just in case there's more to the Great Beyond than I have seen.

5. We need to talk to each other more in this life about death and what lies beyond. I don't mean just getting together at a funeral to reminisce about a loved one's life, nor just discussions over Will's and Powers of Attorney. No, I mean real conversations with people you know and love. There is no reason we shouldn't be able to talk to perfect strangers when it comes to death! I mean, it is the one thing we will all eventually have in common.

We need to talk about what we imagine death to be, share our fears and expectations of death. We should be able to tell the people we love how much we will miss them and why. Dying is the last thing on earth all of us will ever do. Some see this as a great, existential battle where, in the end, death always emerges the victor. I beg to differ. In my experience, death is merely the ticket-taker, ushering us out of this spectacle, as we gain admission to the next Big Show.

4. If you ever consider suicide, don't! Globally, suicide is the 4th leading cause of death among 15- to 29-year-olds. In all, about 1,000 humans kill themselves every day. As indicated before, I have no reason to suspect that suicide is punished in the afterlife, but neither do I have any evidence it's ok to kill yourself.

My only experience with suicide was Leon, of course, and by hearing his account of it, Dr. Adam's mother. Both seemed ok in death, but they also seemed to have a lot of baggage to work through once they died.

The suicide prevention help line is 988. Go ahead and give 'em a call if you're even just musing about killing yourself. You literally have *everything* to lose if you don't.

3. There is never a right time to die. Not a soul I've met was truly ready to go, even the ones who were old or fully at peace with death seemed surprised when it happened and even those who sit with the old and dying, mourn when they're gone.

As we leave this life and go into the next, mature souls painfully peel off the encumbrances of this life, our memories, anguish, our sense of self. For children, that seems easy, yet the death of a child conjures an especially deep grief for those left behind.

In 2021, about 5 million children under the age of 5 perished from the planet. The good news is it used to be much worse. Disease, birth complications and trauma account for most of the child deaths in the world. In first world countries, add in auto accidents and, in the United States, put gun violence high on that list. My point is, life is precious and as a species, we obviously believe this because with each generation we find ways to extend it. Even in our darkest, loneliest moments, life begs us to stay and when, for whatever reason we cannot, the ones we leave behind selfishly mourn our loss.

2. The Universe is good. Like a ginormous, beautiful organism, it would never harm itself and, by extension, all of us within it. The tensions of opposites: birth-death, love-hate, joy-despair etc. are normal within the grand arc of eternity.

There is no reward or punishment in the end for how we navigated these in life, however, I will say this: Life and in turn, death seem to come easier and go more smoothly when one has a clearly imagined idea of where one is headed. It's the folks who've never imagined an afterlife or who failed to recognize the simple beauty of this life, who struggle.

With all its messy contradictions, life really is fascinating, and it has purpose. Whether you're a 101-year-old bi-sexual geezer or a little 5-year-old girl with terminal cancer, your life and death are all part of the plan. We have no idea and no say, at least in this life, as to how that plan evolves. But that shouldn't stop us from questioning, from imagining the itinerary and the ultimate destination.

1. And finally, when I do, at long last, shed this mortal coil, someone please see to it that the Hooligan gets donated to the Kurt Vonnegut Library and Museum in Indianapolis, Indiana. I have no idea how they'll feel about having it, but I sincerely hope someone there will try to reach out to Mr. Vonnegut's soul and tell him what fun I have had with the dang thing!

THE END
(for now)

Acknowledgements

Nobody does anything on their own. My thanks to Penny, my editor, to Abby and to Sian at Between the Lines, my publisher. And to my wife who has no use for my religion but loves me anyway. Here's hoping she's wrong and we really do get to spend eternity together. That would be nice.

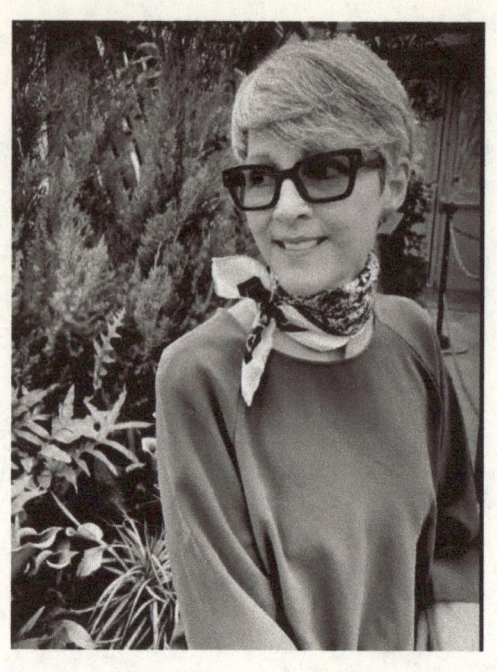

Nan Banks spent most of her lifetime writing professionally, first as a journalist then in corporate communication. Prior to her retirement in 2020, she worked for WYFF-TV in Greenville, SC, for Michelin (both in the US and in France) and for Toyota Motor North America, Inc. now headquartered in Plano, TX. She currently lives with her wife, Jolanta in Asheville, NC.

Death Wish: Tales From Eternity is her first published work of fiction.

Printed in the USA
CPSIA information can be obtained
at www.ICGtesting.com
CBHW012227140324
5384CB00003BA/4